When Johnny Comes Marching Home - With PTSD Trailing Behind Him:

A Book for Those Whose Loved Ones Return from War With PTSD

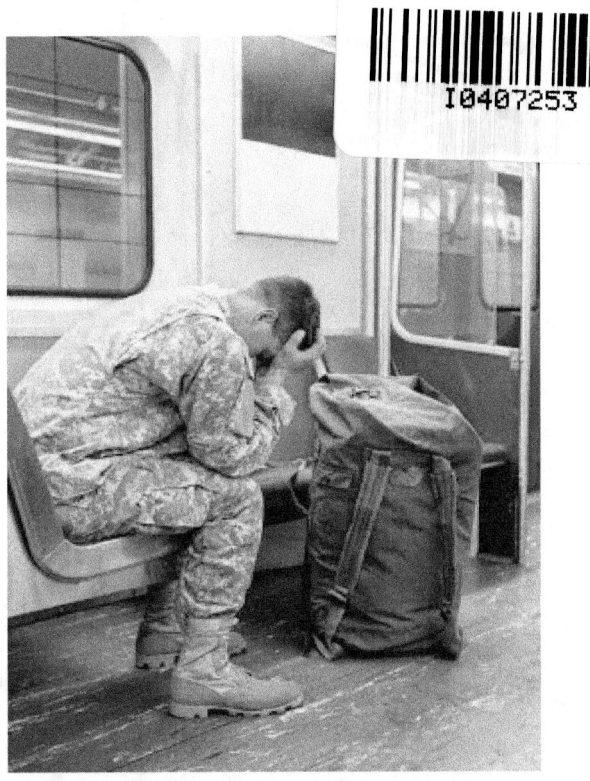

George Lindenfeld, Ph.D.
Diplomate in Clinical Psychology

Table of Content

Praise

"I am a Vietnam Veteran. I did four tours in Vietnam. I didn't realize I had PTSD or even what it was for many years. I had nightmares of the events. I startled easily with loud sounds. I was always looking over my shoulder in fear of the unknown. Intimacy was an issue with me.

"With the encouragement of my wife or perhaps at her insistence, I sought help from the VA. I went through a 12-month program to help me deal with PTSD. I found it to be of little benefit. I continued to have the same issues.

"Finally, my civilian doctor sent me to MindSpa where I met Dr. George Lindenfeld who introduced me to RESET Therapy. It took three sessions till all the trauma faded away. The events were there but they no longer brought out the intense emotions. The nightmares disappeared. It was a new start. It took 50 years but I believe my PTSD is now 100% manageable."

Colonel Retired Dan Cerone

Who Is this Book For?

Our families are struggling with the return of strangers who once were kin. For some of those among us who have sharpened their skills to be warriors, the adjustment back into civilian society becomes a major challenge. The repeated tours abroad make this an even more difficult mission.

Imagine, if you will, having to shift from a place of danger where people die or are maimed while on tour, to a safe world that doesn't understand the dangers just left behind.

My understanding of PTSD is that Mother Nature tried to protect us from having to smell the tiger's breath more than once. Now of course the condition itself is more complex than this, as you will learn in Chapter One of this book. But to begin, I want you to know that we are hard-wired to stay far away from circumstances that created trauma in our lives previously.

Many of you have been told that PTSD cannot be eliminated and that the family needs to learn how to adjust to it. What hasn't been readily revealed to you is the awareness that chronic hyperarousal in your loved one can create secondary PTSD in other members of the family.

It is often difficult for family members to coexist with the new stranger in the home. He or she most likely has insomnia accompanied by flashback experiences and nightmares. A sudden noise in the house can set off a reactive response. This aspect of the condition is referred to as hyperarousal.

I've written this book to be able to direct you and your family to a safe harbor. I will be providing you with varied perspectives from Veterans I've treated throughout this book because I want you to know that a transformation back to normality is possible.

Too many of our servicemen and women have lost hope that an effective change back to their pre-service life is possible. You will be reading stories of Veterans and their families who are struggling to bring productive change back into their world. I will also share stories of those who have become stuck in a continuing world of confusion and fear.

Through this journey, my wish is that you will be better informed of the trials and tribulations that lie before you as you seek to cope with the stranger who returns back to your life. In this sense, information is power as well as wisdom that can be harnessed to steadfastly guide your returning Veteran back into the environment that had been left behind.

I'd like to invite you to visit my webpage for further information at: www.drlindenfeldresettherapy.com. At this site you will find blogs, published articles, additional books, media examples, treatment options and much more. Finally, please consider adding a review of what you think about this book when you complete it.

Acknowledgement

I am forever grateful to those military families who have shared with me their pain and agony regarding their attempts to intervene in a downward spiral for their afflicted servicemen/women. However, even more meaningful is their sharing of joy when the one they love was able to reciprocate by returning love and affection to them once again.

An honorable mention is provided to Brigadier General James Hesson, who so skillfully guided me in my efforts to gain community support for our much-needed study of RESET Therapy with 36-combat Veterans from the greater Sarasota, Florida area. This study will be the first of its kind to scientifically document the effectiveness of this treatment approach.

I extend my appreciation to Dr. Frank Lawlis for his development of the BAUD as well as the basic protocols leading to the later development of RESET Therapy. His wisdom and expertise is truly an enduring foundation that future advances in therapeutic applications can be built upon.

My appreciation to my colleague, Dr. George Rozelle, for providing his 'Brian Mapping' expertise within the context of our study. I would also like to recognize those 'RESET Therapy" Certified

Therapists who participated in remediating the symptoms of PTSD in our Veteran study group. Furthermore, they now offer their skills to those Veterans and civilians within our community at large.

My thanks to Dr. Wayne Rosenfield for his contribution of Veteran vignettes obtained within the context of his involvement in the above referenced study. Furthermore, as our psychometrician, he provided pre-and post-treatment and follow-up assessment to all Veteran participants.

Next, I commend Dr. Michael Sutherland for his statistical expertise in processing all assessment scores that assist us in validating the efficacy of the treatment intervention. I will also express my appreciation to my editor, Dr. James Miller for his physiological wisdom and tireless editing of my written material.

Finally, I extend my thanks to those volunteer Veterans who, without hesitation, have permitted me to utilize their PTSD history and recovery experiences in order to inspire hope in their brother and sisters. This book is dedicated to those who serve or have served to keep us a free people, safe from harm.

Foreword

I am honored to write the forward to Dr. Lindenfeld's newest book, *"When Johnny Comes Marching Home With PTSD Trailing Behind Him.'* As a retired career soldier my interest in Dr. Lindenfeld's RESET therapy treatment began with an article in the local newspaper about a new and novel treatment for Post-Traumatic Stress Disorder (PTSD). Knowing that we are losing 20 veterans per day due to suicide, and that current treatments do not always resolve the problem, I contacted Dr. Lindenfeld to learn more.

I am aware that for service members suffering Post Traumatic Stress (PTS), death for too many is a better solution than constantly reliving the emotions caused by PTS resulting from combat-incurred event(s). For those who don't choose the suicide path, many continue to suffer from the effects of traumatic exposure. Unfortunately, within the family, it manifests itself in broken marriages, emotional scarring of children, alcoholism, homelessness, run-ins with the law, and a myriad of other results caused by the horrific shock they have experienced.

As a soldier, my history includes joining the Minnesota National Guard at age 16. I served 3 combat tours including the Korean War and two Vietnam tours. Even though I ultimately retired, I never left the Army but merely changed a uniform for a suit. As a young soldier, I learned that the most important rule of leadership was to take care of the troops you commanded or supported.

While no longer being in a command position, I still experience the personal commitment to seek out and support ways to end the suffering of those who have served us all so well and so faithfully. Our service members have heard the call as given in President John F. Kennedys inaugural challenge. *"Let every nation know, whether it wishes us well or ill, that we shall pay any price, bear any burden, meet any hardship, support any friend, oppose any foe, in order to assure the survival and the success of liberty"*. In this defense of liberty, many "have borne the burden and paid the price" and often return home changed.

Three times I returned from war zones to a family awaiting my return. I believe I returned unscathed from what I had experienced, but the true judge of my condition on my return was my family. Not all returning service members are, or were as fortunate as I.

Much has been written about our returning service members. However, very little has been written about those at home who await 'Johnny's' return. From this perspective, Dr. Lindenfeld's latest book is specifically focused on those who remained behind. He shares heartbreak and joy in the provided vignettes of those Veterans who have transitioned smoothly or with difficulty or not at all, back into the civilian world.

For the reader, this book offers insight about Post Traumatic Stress (PTS), it's possible causes, and it's potential to infect those who love him/her. Hopefully, through reading this book, those who await a friend or loved one's return, will be better prepared to assist in the Veteran's transition back to pre-deployment life. For me, it's not a disorder but rather, an adaptive change.

This old soldier has chosen not to simply fade away. Rather, I shall serve in the best way I can to support newly emerging therapies that can restore our honored service members to a full and productive life that is free of the emotional scars of war.

I have investigated RESET Therapy including discussing the effects with treated combat Veterans. I have also inquired into the current research investigation with 36 combat Veterans from different eras. Because of my involvement in understanding RESET therapy, I have become a strong advocate for Dr. Lindenfeld's effort to 'end the nightmare of PTSD' and commend this book to all who have a loved one with PTS.

James M. Hesson
Brigadier General, US Army, Retired

Chapter One

What PTSD is & What it Isn't

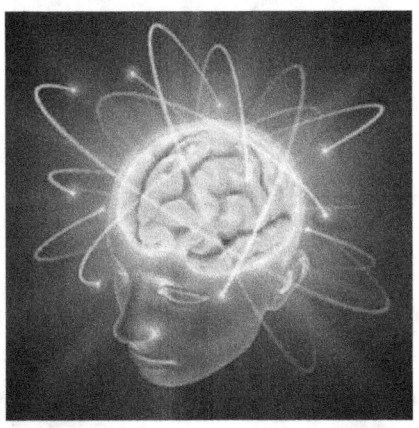

"Unlike simple stress, trauma changes your view of your life and yourself. It shatters your most basic assumptions about yourself and your world — "Life is good," "I'm safe," "People are kind," "I can trust others," "The future is likely to be good" — and replaces them with feelings like "The world is dangerous," "I can't win," "I can't trust other people," or "There's no hope."

Mark Goulston, Post-Traumatic Stress Disorder For Dummies

It is difficult to obtain clarity regarding what happens in the brain and body that causes Post Traumatic Stress Syndrome and why some people apparently develop it and others don't. The United States Department of Veteran's Affairs: National Center for PTSD, tell us that PTSD: "is a mental health problem that some people develop after experiencing or witnessing a life-threatening event, like combat, a natural disaster, a car accident, or sexual assault."

The last thing that those who serve in our military want is anything related to the term, "mental." When coming home from a rotation or for discharge, they may be asked as they depart if they are depressed, etc., to which a "real man" immediately responds in the negative with a loud, "No, Sir!"

Now the way mental health professionals such as psychiatrists, psychologists, etc., go about diagnosing the condition is to go through a checklist of symptoms. You must have two of this type of symptom, one of these, three of these, etc. Causation is not the issue here; whether the symptom is present or not is the primary concern.

When Johnny comes marching home from war and doesn't behave as he did before, you often become aware of this rather quickly; although admittedly, some are inclined to ignore (deny) that something is very wrong.

I'd like to introduce you to Ron LaPointe as he shares his home return story. "In World War II, you got a parade and community support," says Lapointe. "But for Vietnam vets, you got community rejection."

His family, however, embraced him. And after throwing himself into completing his undergraduate studies and attempting to return to his former life, Lapointe flew from Los Angeles to New York to visit his sister, who'd recently moved there.

As he ran through Times Square to catch the next train leaving Grand Central Station for Long Island, a bus backfired. Instinctively, Lapointe dropped, his knees hitting the pavement as his arms came up to cover his head. "That's when I realized there were issues," he says with a sigh.

If only the others Veterans with PTSD could recognize that something is wrong. There are a number of reasons they don't. However, let me complete my dialogue about diagnosis. It is a way to sort people with similar behaviors into groups for numerous reasons including a label by which one can document services rendered.

Thus, if one of the Vets is hearing voices, he is likely to be considered for inclusion in a group of those considered to be schizophrenic. If those voices are suggesting that others are out to get him, he might qualify for a sub-group referred to as paranoid or paranoid schizophrenic.

If he has mood fluctuations he might fit in with the manic/depressive group or perhaps he could qualify for a group called borderline personality disorder. If he does a perimeter check every night before retiring by frequently checking to ensure that the windows and doors are locked throughout the night, he might be considered to be obsessive/compulsive.

I want to clarify to you that diagnosis serves to categorize people that have similar features. Now once that diagnosis has been made, whether it's correct or incorrect, it's difficult to get rid of. Is it any wonder then that our returning warriors would shun being so categorized?

Later, I will introduce you to Robert, who was provided with all of the diagnosis I listed above plus more within the context of his numerous psychiatric hospitalizations. However, the causation of his varied psychiatric symptoms stemmed from his unresolved PTSD.

To state it yet again, diagnosis is used to label folks that share similar symptoms independent of the causation. Let's look at this kind of labelling in the context of military service. For example, in the Navy Sea Bee's the motto is "Can Do." It is not, "I have this kind of weakness, affliction, illness, diagnosis, etc."

Our military members, first responders and members of other male dominated entities are raised, typically from birth, with the *masculine credo*. Now if you're unfamiliar with this term, I'm going to provide you with a definition which, within the context of the military is: a striving for power, assertiveness and dominance.

This makes absolute sense for groups of men who band together for common cause such as honing the skills necessary for killing other people deemed to be the enemy. It can also be a group that arrests people or saves people from fires, etc. The point I make here is that to show weakness of any kind breaks the macho credo or code. Clearly being labeled "mental" in this world is a no-no for those who function within this environment.

It's time for some truth. PTSD is not a "mental illness" at all! Nor is it a character defect or a moral weakness. Rather, it is a systemic hyper-inflammation of the brain initiated by the brain's emotional center called the limbic system. We can actually capture this imagery in picture form.

In other words, when the brain is stuck in a constant state of vigilance, it is unable to return to a resting or balanced state. The body is not designed to be in this circumstance for a prolonged period of time. When this prolongation occurs, things start to go horribly wrong.

This primitive part of our brain, the limbic system, is concerned solely with our survival. It is the initiating agent for responses that we have come to be called the fight, flight, freeze response. Trauma triggers these reactions, setting off alarm bells and whistles in the brain.

The problem is that for many instances of trauma, **when the alarm bell goes off there is no way to shut it down**. It continues to operate every day and every night as though terrible things can still happen at any moment.

Let's revisit Veteran Ron Lapointe's return home. On the plane trip, back to the States, Ron took a few sips of the booze being passed from soldier to soldier. Some men sat quietly, declining to take a swig. Others guzzled gladly at the end of their stint in Vietnam.

Lapointe had landed in the country's central highlands a little more than a year before. On the first day of his deployment in August 1967, the former UCLA international relations student found himself wrapped in a poncho, knee-deep in mud, awaiting orders.

Do you need any 11 Charlies?" (military speak for mortar shells, Lapointe's occupational specialty), one unknown man barked to another. "Do you need any 11 Charlies out there?" he repeated.

But at that moment, louder than even the yelling man and biting rain, Lapointe's intuition told him, "You're going to be OK." Somehow, he remembers, he knew he would survive. And now here he was, heading home.

"Shortly after Lapointe moved back to his family's potato farm in Maine, his mother brought him what she thought was great news. "They're having a celebration for veterans," she told him excitedly. "You should put on your uniform."

Silence.

"Where's your uniform?" "I can't tell you," Lapointe answered. She kept pushing him, and he kept lamenting, "I can't tell you."

"I'll press it for you," she offered. An anguished Lapointe struggled to find a gentle way to tell his mother that she couldn't press a uniform he no longer had.

"Well, where is it?"

Sometime before, Lapointe had walked straight to the barn, taken off his uniform, and burned it in the iron barrel his father used to incinerate the trash. "After the country's response and the effects of war," he says, taking two deep breaths, "I felt ashamed."

After returning home from Vietnam, Ron Lapointe begged his brother to send him his drum kit. Those drums, Lapointe says, "really saved my sanity."

Talking about Vietnam, Lapointe maintains, isn't going to help. "I don't want to sit in a room of vets, particularly combat vets, and share war stories," he says. "Why relive something you don't want to relive?"

Herein lies at least one of the reasons why our returning Veterans don't want to relive their traumatic experiences. Talking about it re-triggers the bodily reactions that are part of the recollections of the trauma.

These memories have become permanently fixed in nerve cells (neuronal) in a network of the brain that repeatedly fires when triggered. In the body, it feels as though the trauma is actually happening again in the immediate moment.

It's like your serviceman was magically transported back to Fallujah with all of the scenes, smells, sounds, heat or cold, and horrors occurring before him as though he has entered a virtual reality world. In his mind, he is back there, repeating the event unchanged each time it is triggered.

So, here's another truth (mine) – traditional psycho-therapy based on talk and logic can't touch the "angry cobra" that lives in the emotional center (limbic system) of the brain. Get close to it – threaten it in any way – and it will instinctively try to sink its fangs into you.

I'll tell you how I came to adopt this startling and scary imagery. While in Asheville, North Carolina, I did subcontracting work with a company that provided Diagnostic Intake material by licensed psychiatrists and psychologists to the Veterans Administration. This was done in order to determine disability ratings for PTSD or TBI (Traumatic Brain Injury) in Veterans who applied for disability benefits.

I remember asking an older, well-spoken Veteran what it was like having PTSD inside of him. Here's what he said: "Inside of my brain is a pissed-off cobra, hood flared, ready to strike at anything, anyone who dares to come close to it!"

Wow, the hair on my skin stood alert. I had never heard anyone describe it so succinctly. I used and expanded upon this startling imagery thereafter.

For example, I added the idea that the cobra's poison could be transmitted to those who are or become emotionally involved with their marine or soldier, airman or sailor. In this way, other family members come to develop Secondary PTSD.

Trauma therapists can be poisoned by listening to and empathizing with the PTSD soldier. Physicians and nurses can absorb the poison through daily contact with the manifestations of physical as well as emotional trauma in their patients. In cases of this type, it is called compassion fatigue, burnout and ultimately, PTSD.

It is understandable why others are repelled by the carrier of such poison. As those around her pull away, the Veteran slides into a transition of alienation, isolation and disconnection. Did you know that 9% of homeless Veterans are female?

I told you earlier that I would share Robert's story with you. Robert served honorably in the Vietnam War as a gunner who was thrust into horrific experiences that are difficult for a human being to imagine. He has suffered for nearly 50 years from the after effects of this experience, unable to shake the traumatic memories that have haunted him.

He has struggled to cope with a sleep disorder referred to as insomnia, drug use and overwhelming anxiety complicated further by misdiagnosis, unsuccessful therapy, multiple hospitalizations, and numerous medications that left him numb and devoid of his personality. He is like tens of thousands of other vets who continue to suffer in silence.

In Robert's Diagnostic Intake he revealed that, "Things would flare-up and I would get into fights. I did drugs. I stopped taking my medications because I was still having flashbacks." His wife reported that her husband was quite mean toward her and that she was at her wit's end trying to deal with his endless anger and rage.

Robert joined the Marines in exchange for having criminal charges against him dropped in court. His juvenile years were troublesome and he was frequently in trouble with the law for minor violations. It was not unusual during this period for judges to offer options such as the choice of jail time or enlistment.

From Camp Pendleton, he was deployed to Vietnam and a couple of weeks later he was called into combat as a mortar gunman. In one gruesome instance,

Robert described how he was directed to help about 20 wounded Marines in the field aboard a chopper and then he had to collect the bodies of those that died whose remains lay in the field.

> "We packed all the bodies in a pile as we were fighting and a round came in and hit them. There were body parts everywhere. We had to gather them up. I've had lots of flashbacks of picking up the pieces."

Another incident involved firing rounds of white phosphorous on houses after they had tried to evacuate the inhabitants.

> "There were many people that just wouldn't come out. When we hit the houses all the kids and others started coming out. Some were killed and some died later. Word was that all of them died. That has haunted me for years and years.

> "After I got back from Vietnam I had flashbacks and nightmares. For 15 to 20 years I was nothing but an alcoholic and a drug addict. I would bolt upright from sleep at night terrified because I thought I was in combat."

His flashbacks started a few months after returning. Some of the triggers were the smells of gunpowder, burning meat or decomposition and fireworks. Robert was hospitalized over 30 times after being diagnosed by the VA as being paranoid schizophrenic and a psychopath. I carefully reviewed DSM-IV criteria for PTSD within the context of this patient's symptomatology in contrast with criteria necessary for the diagnosis of paranoid schizophrenia.

It became glaringly apparent to me that this patient had been misdiagnosed and provided with medications that are used for those who are chronically psychotic. Tracing his history thoroughly, including his war experiences, led me to believe that the primary causative factor for his erratic and at times bizarre behavior was his exposure to traumatic war events. The absence of structure in his developmental history as well as the death of his mother when he was a teenager certainly increased his vulnerability.

Given his diagnosis and negative prior experiences with traditional psychotherapy and medication, I chose to utilize RESET Therapy as an initial treatment of choice. After explaining that this was an experimental treatment, I carefully tuned the device's sound to resonate (connect) with one of his trauma targets.

Robert was provided with a 15-minute intervention utilizing this neuromodulation treatment. He was asked to bring up in his mind the memory and emotions that he had previously avoided at all cost. On his return visit one week later, Robert reported that,

> "I was thinking about the event and all but it seemed more peaceful. I haven't had any nightmares or flashbacks compared to previously having them 2 to 3 times per week."

His wife reported that her husband had done some work on the car rather than just sitting despondently in the house.

> "Now he talks again and is carrying on conversations. He didn't do that before. He would just lay in bed with a dark look on his face eating and watching TV all the time. His communication is getting better and he is getting back to the way he used to be.

> "He helps with the chores. The very first treatment he had was like a miracle. He went home, slept well, didn't jerk awake, didn't jump up awake slamming, screaming, looking like someone was going to kill him."

Robert perceived that he was doing better with his Vietnam issues and consequently, he was encouraged to test his limits by watching war movies focusing on this era. He was seen in follow-up one week later and reported that:

> "I watched a war story and it didn't bother me at all. When I wake up I feel great! I don't argue over any little things anymore. I was talking with a guy about Vietnam and it didn't bother me."

His wife noted that, "He hasn't been having any nightmares and doesn't jerk anymore at night. Overall he is improving but I'm concerned about his gambling problem."

Robert selected his next target, which, at his wife's insistence, was focused on his urge to gamble. On his return the following week he reported that, "I don't want to play anymore. The charge in it for me is gone."

His wife added that, "His whole attitude is changed. He seems to be doing marvelously well." A final therapy target was selected which consisted of his resentment towards his father for favoring his older sister and brother.

"My father met me at the airport when I came back from Vietnam. That was the first time he actually ever seemed to be glad to see me. I was close to my mom but she died when I was 15. I probably never got over her death."

In his final appointment, he relayed that he was feeling better about this matter and was now able to go with things on his own. He has been followed since therapy through telephone contact as well as email. His PTSD has remained in remission for well over four years at the time of the writing of this chapter.

Robert's case illustrates the complexity frequently seen in Vietnam era patients with chronic PTSD and other accompanying issues. In Robert's case, this included gambling and family of origin issues. With those who have experienced trauma during their developmental years, I have found recovery to occur but not as rapidly as when the causative factor is primarily war related.

Indeed, a key authority in the field, Dr. Bessel van der Kolk in Psychiatric Annals, May 2005, noted that the term "Complex Trauma describes the experience of multiple, chronic and prolonged developmentally adverse traumatic events, most often of an interpersonal nature (eg. Sexual or physical abuse, war, community violence) and early life onset."

Taking this a step further, a blog (Healing Resources.info) contains a post entitled: "Trauma, Attachment, and Stress Disorders: Rethinking and Reworking Developmental Issues." Within this post, the author notes that:

"There is a correlation between early trauma and resiliency or vulnerability to highly stressful experiences later in life. People who have been traumatized as infants and young children are more at risk for traumatic experiences later in life. In helping people who have become traumatized, we don't need to be neuroscientists but we do need to use interventions that change the brain.

". . . Trauma and loss are parts of life. It is not what happens to us but how we react to it that determines whether or not a life-threatening experience or a series of less intense experiences will, in fact, be traumatizing. The more vulnerable the organism, the more it is at risk for the neural dysregulation that can follow traumatic experiences.

"Whether dysregulation follows an intense event described with symptoms of PTSD or a seemingly benign event or series of events with symptoms like depression, anxiety or relationship disorders, emotionally traumatizing events contain three common elements:

- It was unexpected;
- The person was unprepared; and
- There was nothing the person could do to prevent it from happening." ("Trauma, Attachment, and Stress disorders: Developmental Issues,")

It does appear, based on rather comprehensive scientific inquiry, that developmental traumatic experiences increase vulnerability to the emergence of PTSD in combat related situations. However, this is a contributing factor that is not the sole causative agent. It seems likely that those sensitized to trauma in their developmental years are at increased risk for combat incurred PTSD from their battlefield experiences.

In this first chapter, I have told you that PTSD is not a mental condition but, rather, an instinctive reaction from a primitive part of our brain that doesn't respond to talk, love, empathy or any other form of caring emotion. The snake wants only one thing – to survive at all cost.

I've described a 'macho' male culture that frowns on labels such as 'mental' and 'illness.' I've discussed the purpose of diagnoses and noted that it has absolutely nothing to do with causation. I've given you case examples of transitions gone awry with decades of suffering thereafter.

Most importantly, I've defined PTSD as a systemic hyper-inflammation of the brain initiated by the brain's emotional center called the limbic system. I've explained that this occurs when the brain becomes locked into a defensive, self-protective mode that is unable to return to its natural state of balance.

I want you to see what it looks like when the cobra's hood is flared, fangs ready to attack followed by how it appears when the cobra's fangs are at rest.

PTSD RECALL OF TRAUMA
PRE-RESET THERAPY

GREEN = NORMAL, RED = EXCESSIVE

Montage: Laplacian   EEG ID: Startdate 25-SEP-2015 3.001.01_EC GR SN:060448

Z Scored FFT Summary Information

| Delta | Theta | Alpha | Beta | High Beta |

Absolute Power

RECALL OF TRAUMA
POST-RESET THERAPY

Montage: Laplacian   EEG ID: 6.001.01_EC

Z Scored FFT Summary Information

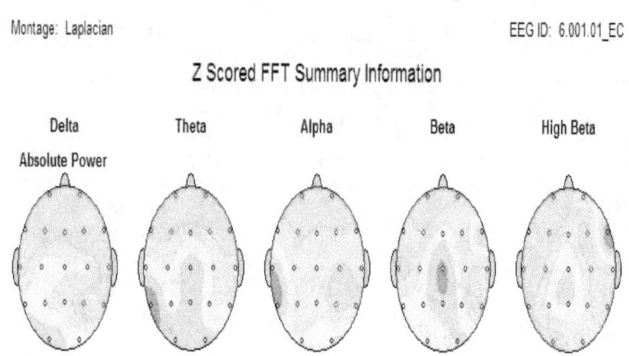

They say that a picture is worth more than a thousand words. Upon looking at the first image provided, my colleague, Dr. George Rozelle spontaneously said: "It looks like his brain is on fire." I have consequently used this in a paper George and I coauthored as well as in the title of my second book.

To see the qEEG displays in full color, please visit my webpage at: www.drlindenfeldresettherapy.com. At the Home Page, scroll down to the media button and click on media. You will find academia which will bring up my paper: Brain On Fire.

The red/orange in the pre-treatment qEEG image represents the Veteran's hyper-inflammation state when triggering his selected trauma target. This same technique is utilized post-treatment. This one is free of the neuro-inflammation associated with PTSD. You'll learn more about Corporal Wade Risha later in this book (the images above are his) and how his life has changed.

I don't want you to be confused by these images so I'll briefly explain what they're all about. When brain wave electricity is measured, usually by the neurologist, it is broken down into different groupings going from very slow waves (Delta) to very active waves (High Beta). The display you are viewing reveal the breakdown of the waves in each of the varied EEG domains all produced by one person over a specific period of time.

I show you these images early in this book because I want you, the family, to know that transformative change is possible for your loved one. I want you to rekindle hope once again if it has become lost in your despair. Listen with caution to those who tell you that your son/daughter needs to be medicated and psycho-therapized for the rest of their life. I say PTSD can be RESET. The cobra can be quieted!

The following chapters are designed to provide you, the concerned family member, with safe passage to guide you through the pitfalls you are likely to encounter on this critical journey. Each chapter will include Veterans transitions when thing go horribly wrong. My goal is to provide guidance from a world of nightmare to one of reality, stability and the capacity to give and receive love and affection from others. Keep this foremost in your mind as you read further.

References

Trauma, Attachment, and Stress disorders: Developmental Issues. http://www.healing resources .info/ trauma_attachment_stress_disorders .htm

Chapter Two

Stuck in the Mud

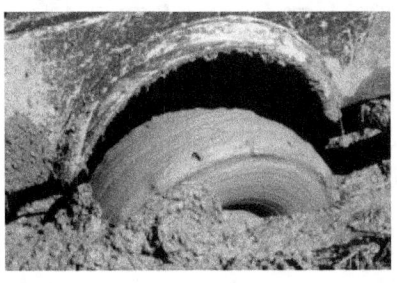

"How strange
that the nature of life
is change,
yet the nature of human beings
is to resist change.
And how ironic
that the difficult times
we fear might ruin us
are the very ones
that can break us open
and help us blossom
into who we were meant to be."

**Elizabeth Lesser, Broken Heart: How
Difficult Times Can Help Us Grow**

A *New York Times Magazine* article written by C. J. Shivers entitled: "The Fighter" was published on January 1, 2017. The subheading of the article was: "The Marine Corps Taught Sam Siatta How to Shoot. The War in Afghanistan Taught Him How to Kill. Nobody Taught Him How to Come Home."

I will provide you with brief excerpts in line with the constraints of copyright laws. My intent is to follow the topic of this chapter however, I suggest that you read this piece in its entirety.

****

. . . He also had no clear reason to have entered someone else's home, no motive that prosecutors would be able to point to at trial. . . His former company commander would later tell a trial judge that of the 388 troops he led in Afghanistan, Siatta was the man the militants feared most.

Major Scott A. Cuomo . . . said Siatta was a solid Marine in combat – a gifted marksman trusted by his peers, invaluable in firefights and deserving of gratitude, not incarceration.

In his diary, Siatta wrote the following: '. . . I hope my family recognizes me when I get back, and I hope they understand I've changed but only through the acts of self preservation. My mind cannot be healed from the horrors of war. I hope they understand.'

He wrote further that: '. . . I go to sleep every night knowing that I have the blood of so many on my hands and no amount of soap could ever wash these stains away.'

When his battalion returned to Camp Lejeune, his mother . . . noticed that: . . . (Siatta) did not sleep at night and did not leave his bed most of the day. He spoke very little.

Upon returning to his family home he contacted his former girlfriend. . . Looking at him after their long separation, she sensed that something troubled him. She tried drawing him out. . . That night they made love. 'I felt our old connection' she said. Immediately after, Siatta withdrew.

As she lay beside him, he reached for a blanket and wrapped it tightly around his body, with all his limbs tucked inside. ("The Fighter - The New York Times,")

****

Behavioral indicators were evident in the above story that I want family members to be aware of. Certainly time-lag is a factor that requires adjustment. However, after a reasonable time, most people adapt to the time change. If Johnny doesn't, it is likely that we are looking at insomnia, a hallmark feature found in PTSD.

It might be worthwhile to follow his sleeping pattern for a night or two. Is he up frequently? Are there nightmares that occur? You're gathering information about your loved one. Is he able to talk about his experiences overseas? Is Johnny using alcohol, marijuana, etc., in order to self-medicate?

While away from you, things and events in your world progressed leaving Johnny behind while his world went in a different direction. A world of protect and defend. Perhaps gradually you can help catch him up to what has transpired back home. This might be done causally at opportune times in a natural way. It's rather difficult, for example, for Johnny to remember that a cousin entered high school when your Veteran was avoiding ambushes while on patrol.

As more of our troops come home, Veterans who have successfully made the transition back to veteran life are volunteering to assist a recently returned Vet to successfully negotiate the transition. If possible, check out if this is a possibility prior to your loved one's return. Setting up this connection in advance can make the difference between a successful or a failed transition. A successful life as opposed to one that becomes, "stuck in the mud."

Remember, the military functions as a family in its own right. The support came from those he fought with, served with, endured hardships with. They lived together, shared military-speak with each other, ate lousy food together, lived the danger of modern warfare together.

During her service, there was no time off. No weekends to relax. No sweetheart to squeeze. No safe place to rest. A patrol is fraught with danger including being among a population that may wish and pray for your loved one's death.

When she traveled, she may have been vulnerable to mortar attack, roadside bombs or car bombs. Perhaps, you weren't aware that on December 3, 2016, Defense Secretary Ashton B. Carter said that the Pentagon would open all combat jobs to women.

"There will be no exceptions," Mr. Carter said at a news conference. He added, "They'll be allowed to drive tanks, fire mortars and lead infantry soldiers into combat. They'll be able to serve as Army Rangers and Green Berets, Navy SEALs, Marine

Corps infantry, Air Force para-jumpers and everything else that was previously open only to men."

"The groundbreaking decision overturns a longstanding rule that had restricted women from combat roles, even though women have often found themselves in combat in Iraq and Afghanistan over the past 14 years.

"It is the latest in a long march of inclusive steps by the military, including racial integration in 1948 and the lifting of the ban on gay men and lesbians serving openly in the military in 2011. The decision this week will open about 220,000 military jobs to women." (Rosenberg & Philipps, 2015)

When he fights, someone might die. This could be the enemy, an acquaintance or a close friend. Each morning when he arises, he likely wonders if this one will be his last. Alternatively, he may sense that he will make it back. Whatever his perception, the adrenaline rush is pumping in high drive, twenty-four seven.

When he finally leaves combat and returns home, the people he's known are unfamiliar to him. Their sounds, smells and behaviors are peculiar at first. You see, like any predator, he's come to rely on his animal senses to stay alive. This protective demeanor makes it difficult to let down his guard and assume the role of civilian again.

When it comes to intimacy, sure, he can let down his guard briefly. But immediately after, he wraps himself in that blanket again like Sam Siatta did with his sweetheart. It doesn't have to be a physical blanket. We all have to capacity to put up an emotional shield to keep others distant when we feel threatened. The problem is that some can't take the shield down!

Plan on his not engaging well with the family at first. You might almost expect this. However, if this continues over an excessive amount of time, see this as his being stuck in the transition process. For many of our younger active duty personnel, they yearn for their next rotation, not so much to be in harm's way again but, to get back to the world they've know.

This is both a dangerous as well as exciting world. For those who served in the Iraq and Afghanistan conflicts 47% reported serving with a comrade that had been killed. The following article brings this point home.

"Exposure to casualties also had an effect on the emotional well-being of many veterans. Veterans who suffered their own injuries, or experienced the death or serious injuries of others, were more than twice as likely (54% to 22%) to say they had undergone an emotionally traumatic or distressing event during their service than those not exposed to casualties. Veterans exposed to casualties were also more likely to say, by 42% to 27%, that they suffered from post-traumatic stress." (comments, 2015)

All of his old civilian patterns require rehearsal again. Integrating back into the civilian world takes practice and courage. If unmarried, divorced or separated, dating is yet another challenge. Talking to a civilian is awkward when all you've done for seven months or more is to talk military-speak.

The military experience has grown more intense and the likelihood of engaging in combat has increased. This is due to the nature of our current conflicts as well as the diminishing number of people who currently serve. This figure has dropped significantly in the past fifty years from 3.1 million in 1966 to 1.3 million in today's all-voluntary force. This constitutes less than 1% of all U.S. adults. (comment, 2016)

He may perceive your comments and attitude erroneously perceiving that he's a misshaped cog that not fitting well into the family gear. It is not at all unusual for him to believe that he is unwanted or unneeded. Expect that when this occurs, he will be inclined to withdraw and self-isolate.

Dealing with the lingering stress that accompanies him home is a given. Remember that he has slept with his weapon near to him. It now feels awkward to be without it. His emotional brain feels vulnerable and in harm's way without the protection of his rifle. He misses the guys ribbing him, the master sergeant setting him straight, the sense of someone protecting his six (military-speak for his back).

Anger is another manifestation of the residual stress that he's lived with over the tour. You see, in order to kill the enemy, you must depersonalize him. He who is the enemy is the one that maimed his buddy by placing an IED along the road or ambushed his patrol and killed his closest friend.

Keeping that anger allows his to keep his senses razor sharp. That's what helped him to survive. Now that he's home, the cobra inside his emotional center doesn't know the difference. So, who is he to take his anger out on now? Could it be his wife or his children or perhaps, he might be putting himself in harm's way?

When Johnny comes home you may be struck by changes in his demeanor. Whereas once he was a calm and unexcitable person, he is now quite impulsive or may be thrill seeking. His risk-taking behaviors may seem to take place particular at times when he is feeling down.

One Operation Desert Storm Veteran arrived early for his appointment at an office in a busy metropolitan area. He propped the door open with his body, guiding a very heavy-looking bicycle into the office waiting room. The receptionist directed him to store the bicycle in the narrow corridor behind her work area. Because he was early, he was invited to the office permitting us to chat informally before getting to the issue at hand.

****

Making small talk, he was asked if it was scary riding his bicycle on these busy streets. 'No, I love it' he said. 'I ride on the bike lane, close to the traffic.'

That's not scary? 'Not at all. I love the excitement. It gives me a rush. I like the danger of trucks and cars zipping past me; the loud engines, everything. There was a big truck with one of those old, growling engines. It reminded me of the military trucks. And when I smell the exhaust...Man, it's like being in convoy. I love it!

'Do you have a helmet? 'Nope. I go everywhere on my bike. And I miss it when

I'm not out riding. It's like I need to do it'.
'And you like the danger?' 'Hell, yeah. It's an
adrenaline high.'

****

To appreciate the proportion of our veterans'
transitional issues I will utilize an April 2014 article
by Michele A. Flournoy entitled: "We aren't doing
enough to help veterans transition to civilian life."
The author notes that:

"Over the past 13 years, roughly 2.4 million active
and reserve members of the U.S. armed forces have
left military service and returned to civilian life. In
the next four to five years, another million, most of
whom are post-9/11 veterans, will make this
transition.

"The transition from uniformed duty to civilian status
is not just a change of jobs, it's a change in virtually
every aspect of life: their careers, responsibilities,
jobs, homes, communities, lifestyle, health care,
training and more. If service members have families,
the transition will also mean big changes for spouses
and children, maybe even more so because these
family members largely have no access to continuing
support from the Department of Veterans Affairs.

"Not surprisingly, half of the respondents in the poll
said their readjustment to civilian life was difficult.

They cited various reasons, from struggles in finding a good job to inadequate assistance from the government. What is striking about this data is how multidimensional the problem is — showing how difficult it is to solve.

". . . One crucial area of disconnect between veterans' expectations and reality is their prospects for civilian employment. Sixty-six percent of the veterans polled believed they have the education and skills to be competitive in today's job market; 81 percent thought their skills would translate well to the civilian job market; and 62 percent thought employers would see military service as an advantage.

"These high expectations contrast with what many post-9/11 veterans are experiencing: Whereas the jobless rate for all U.S. veterans was just 6.9 percent in October 2013 — slightly lower than for the overall population — the unemployment rate for veterans who have served since 9/11 stood at 10 percent." ("'I miss Iraq every day,'")

I now shift the discussion to a topic that is quite unnerving but must be discussed. For some returning home, they bring emotional and physical damage imposed on them by their own. The issue of Military Sexual Violence (MST) must be brought into the light of day as it may apply to your returning loved one.

This is a topic that most want to avoid but in a military environment (particularly in combat zones) access to typical sexual interactions is frequently blocked. Therefore, a simple truth need be shared: most rapists force victims to have sex because they (rapists) want sex. It has nothing to do with power, control, etc. The military rapist feels deprived of a sexual outlet. The intensity of engagement in combat likely heightens their sexual arousal.

"Sexual offenders of all ages prefer young victims. Even elderly offenders target 15-year-olds the most. Also, men who commit sexual assault tend to be considerably older than men who commit other types of violent crimes.

"The relatively high rate of sexual offending by older men is likely due to the fact that they have become less attractive with age while their sexual attraction to young people is undiminished. The men and women they find most attractive are not attracted to them. Some of them use force to get their way. ("To Rape is to Want Sex, Not Power | Quillette,")

A study of the incidence of sexual assault reported by both pre- and post-9/11 female veterans is generally consistent with what has been previously reported among female veteran.

". . . approximately 20% to 43% reporting experiencing sexual assault while in the military. . .The prevalence of sexual assault during military service in pre-9/11 female veterans was particularly high with almost half reporting being the victim of sexual assault during their military service." (Kintzle et al., 2015)

The official definition of MST used by the VA is: "Psychological trauma, which in the judgment of a VA mental health professional, resulted from a physical assault of a sexual nature, battery of a sexual nature, or sexual harassment which occurred while the Veteran was serving on active duty or active duty for training. Sexual harassment is defined as 'repeated, unsolicited verbal or physical contact of a sexual nature which is threatening in character.'

"In more concrete terms, MST includes any sexual activity where you were involved against your will. You may have been physically forced into sexual activities. Or, no physical force may have been used but you were coerced or pressured into sexual activities.

"For example, you may have been threatened with negative consequences for refusing to cooperate. Or it may have been suggested that you would get faster promotions or better treatment in exchange for sex. These are all signs of MST.

"If these experiences occurred while you were on active duty or active duty for training, they are considered to be MST." (Kintzle et al., 2015) For example, a female (Anonymous, United States Army) reported the following:

****

I joined the military at 18 because my mother was sick. She died when I was 19yrs old in A.I.T. Two months later I was sent to Korea within being there a month I was raped by a upper ranking soldier. I was already devastated by the death of my mother this just pushed me over the edge.

After trying to cope for a few weeks I couldn't so I took an overdose of percocet. At the hospital I found out I was pregnant with his child. I was horrified. I didn't know what to do.

In the hospital I informed my female Sargent and she told me to keep quiet no one will believe me. She then told me to go off post in Korea and find a abortions doctor. Abortion is illegal in Korea and they wouldn't allow me on a plane until I was 6 months. I had never felt so alone. I gave birth to her and my family would not allow me to give her up.

She is now 13 and thriving I am a mental case and dying. Its hard enough seeing your attackers face everyday, but even harder losing your life and having no help. They did DNA and it was his. He pays a few dollars a month but he still gets to live his life.

The military refuses to acknowledge my assault. I suppose if it didn't happen this child must be a ghost. I struggle everyday to pay bills, to eat, to care for this child, I have no car, I'm a prisoner serving time. I need help. I was only 19yrs old, what about me?? (mydutytospeak, 2016)

****

The point I am making here is that factors other than combat incidents can produce PTSD in your loved one related to his/her military service. Please listen to what your child, sibling, companion, wife/husband has to say. And if they say nothing but appear distant and cut off, see this as a sign that experiences likely occurred that cannot be expressed in words at this time.

A final comment on this topic, please don't be so naïve that you think that MST only occurs to around one in five females who serve or have served. Information from the US Department of Veteran Affairs PTSD: National Center for PTSD, Men and Sexual Trauma reports that:

"At least 1 out of every 10 (or 10%) of men in our country have suffered from trauma as a result of sexual assault. Like women, men who experience sexual assault may suffer from depression, posttraumatic stress disorder (PTSD), and other emotional problems as a result.

"However, because men and women have different life experiences due to their different gender roles, emotional symptoms following trauma can look different in men than they do in women. A Pentagon report notes that:

"Sexual assault is alarmingly common in the U.S. military, and more than half of the victims are men. According to the Pentagon, thirty-eight military men are sexually assaulted every single day.

"These are the stories you never hear—because the culprits almost always go free, the survivors rarely speak, and no one in the military or Congress has done enough to stop it." ("Men and Sexual Trauma - PTSD,")

****

On the morning of September 20, two weeks before the warship was due in port, three men ambushed Stovey in a remote storage area of the ship, where he'd been sent to get supplies. They threw a black hood over his head, strangled and sodomized him, then left him for dead on a stack of boxes. Stovey told no one. He was certain that his attackers, whose faces he hadn't glimpsed, would kill him if he did. He hid in a bathroom until he could contain his panic and tolerate the pain. Then he quietly returned to his post.

Stovey says he might have killed himself were it not for his father's imminent arrival. The timing of the visit was "almost a miracle," he says. "When I saw him, it was the most safe feeling I'd ever felt in my whole life."

Father and son spent the next five days on board ship, almost certainly being watched by the three attackers. "I just kept it inside," Stovey says in a low voice. "I couldn't tell him. ("'Son, Men Don't Get Raped,'")

****

"Those who sexually assault men or boys differ in a number of ways from those who assault only females. Boys are more likely than girls to be sexually abused by strangers or by authority figures in organizations such as schools, the church, or athletics programs.

"Those who sexually assault males usually choose young men and male adolescents (the average age is 17 years old) as their victims and are more likely to assault many victims, compared to those who sexually assault females. Perpetrators often assault young males in isolated areas where help is not readily available. For instance, a perpetrator who assaults males may pick up a teenage hitchhiker on a remote road or find some other way to isolate his intended victim.

"As is true about those who assault and sexually abuse women and girls, most perpetrators of males are men. Specifically, men are perpetrators in about 86 out of every 100 (or 86%) of male victimization cases." ("Men and Sexual Trauma - PTSD,") Also, as reported in the US Department of Veteran Affairs PTSD, Military Sexual Trauma:

"Prevalence estimates obtained from these screening data have remained generally consistent since then, and as of 2008, these clinical populations numbered 48,106 women and 43,693 men. The populations are similar in size, despite the lower prevalence of MST among men, because VHA treats so many more men than women." ("Military Sexual Trauma - v20n2. pdf,")

It's now time to shift gears to provide you with other important information related to your loved one's transition efforts. Let's begin with the likelihood that your Veteran will likely be unaware of changes in personal finances after leaving the military.

This will include the probable necessity to take a pay cut to enter into civilian employment. Furthermore, it may take much longer than anticipated to secure a position that would fit in with prior military training. Then the issues of medical insurance, cost of living, applying for medical benefits, etc., come on like a fast-moving thunderstorm. Sites such as The Military Wallet and The Military Guide can be quite helpful in this regard.

Many of our newly released Veterans incorrectly estimate the competitiveness of the job market. Often, this requires your loved one to "suck it up" and take a position on the lower rung of the ladder to begin the steps necessary to advance. For some, this is humiliating and pride interferes with reality. Be there to support him/her with these hurdles to compete this obstacle course successfully. Some excellent pointers are available in the following 2017 blog:

"No matter what you do when you leave the military, it's going to involve salesmanship. . . Advocating for why a subordinate deserves a promotion, getting buy-in from a team for a plan of action . . However, the sale that will be most essential in your transition will also be the most difficult for you — you'll have to sell yourself.

". . . "It's up to you to tell them your story — you need to practice over and over again, because it's a new skill set, and something you never had to do in the military." That's why it's so vital to get your reps in and get comfortable with this aspect as it is not going away."

". . . Self-knowledge emerged as the overriding theme in what was most critical in the transition to a civilian career. Whether you realize it or not, your military service is an enormous part of your identity — an identity you'll need to refine and expand as you enter the next chapter of your life. Your ability to be challenging and honest with yourself will make the most critical difference in narrowing your job search . . . and finding a job that will make you fulfilled." (Nassiri, 2017)

Another online resource for veterans to find the right civilian job_is available at Military One Source. ("Land a Civilian Job After Military Service,") Using your computer helps to better target potential opportunities. Important advice is available at the above source such as:

- **"Clarify your skills and strengths.** First, get a copy of your Verification of Military Experience and Training through the Department of Defense. ("vmet_instructions.pdf,") Then, think about how your strengths and your skills could be applied in a work setting. If you're drawing a blank, a career assessment could point you to career fields that are a good match. Your installation's transition office can set you up with a test at no cost.

- **"Check your qualifications and licenses.** Your military licenses or certifications might not translate to a civilian equivalent. Check out the Army's Credentialing Opportunities Online website to learn how to market your military license to a civilian employer." (Absher,)

Another focus for returning Veterans to consider is the educational route. This can be for specific job training such as that available through a technical school track. Other focus may be more academic in nature.

1. **Decide whether to try to change your career path** — If your military career path doesn't align with your ultimate goals,

consider changing directions. Your unit's career planner or career counselor can provide more information on changing your career field.

2. **Consider assessment testing** — Don't wait until retirement time to test your skills. Your installation military and family support center, Transition Assistance Program or Army Career and Alumni Program can help you find out if you're best suited to be a prima ballerina or a stockbroker.

3. **Pursue your education** — Education is a major benefit of military service. College degrees and military leadership courses can help build a solid resume.

4. **Learn to communicate** - Volunteer to give briefs to commanders on your unit's activities or participate in any other public speaking you can. Sell your unit's accomplishments and build skills you can use to land yourself a civilian job later.

5. **Find a mentor** — You're not the first to transition from a military to a civilian career, so use the knowledge in your community. Find a military mentor who can help you find the right schools or advise you how to

advance your career. A civilian mentor in your field can help you keep abreast of trends outside the military including information that can help guide your career inside the military.

6. **Volunteer** —Volunteering can help you get your foot in the door in the civilian world, especially if you're taking a drastic turn with your occupational choice.

7. **Obtain required licenses and certifications** — Many military certifications don't transfer readily to the civilian world (bummer) but it may be easier to attain a corresponding civilian license or certification while you're still in the military. For more information on civilian certification and licensing, visit the Army's Credentialing Opportunities On-Line.

Summary

This chapter began with segments of a *New York Times Magazine* article focused on the topic of our combat Veterans being poorly prepared for their transition back into the civilian world. This was followed with an uncomfortable topic that is generally considered to be a taboo in our society.

This issue of Military Sexual Trauma (MST) must be faced head on particularly with females now serving in all positions including combat related roles. With estimates ranging around 20 to 43%. With men, the estimates range from 1.1% to around 10%.

A brief discussion was provided pertaining to employment as well as educational opportunities. As a family member, consider checking resources for your returning service member. I'd advise starting with a VA office closest to you. I suggest this as our younger returning Veterans, particularly those with PTSD, are inclined to avoid governmental entities. Find out beforehand what educational and employment opportunities are available locally.

The next chapter focuses on those 30 to 50% who experience difficulty in their transition. Among these are those with Complex PTSD as well as combat related trauma issues.

References

Absher, J. Army Credentialing Opportunities On Line Army COOL http://www.military.com /education/finding-a-school/army-credentia ling-opportunities-on-line-army-cool.html

comment, G. L. a. (2016, November 11). Profile of U.S. veterans is changing dramatically as their ranks decline. http://www.pewresearch .org/fact-tank/2016/11/11/profile-of-u-s-veterans-is-changing-dramatically-as-their-ranks-decline/

comments, B. D. (2015, May 22). Memorial Day: About half of veterans of post-9/11 wars served with someone who was killed. http://www.pewresearch.org/fact-tank/2015/05/22/about-half-of-veterans-of-post-911-wars-served-with-someone-who-was-killed/

"I miss Iraq every day." http://www.washingtonpost.com/posttv/national/i-miss-iraq-every-day/2014/03/28/e1640746-b5f4-11e3-bab2-b9602293021d_video.html

Kintzle, S., Schuyler, A. C., Ray-Letourneau, D., Ozuna, S. M., Munch, C., Xintarianos, E., … Castro, C. A. (2015). Sexual trauma in the military: Exploring PTSD and mental health care utilization in female veterans. *Psychological Services, 12*(4), 394–401. https://doi.org/10.1037/ser0000054

Land a Civilian Job After Military Service. http://www.militaryonesource.mil/deployment-and-transition/separating-from-the-military?content_id=281376

Men and Sexual Trauma - PTSD: National Center for PTSD. http://www.ptsd.va.gov/public/types/violence/men-sexual-trauma.asp

Military Sexual Trauma - v20n2.pdf. http://www.ptsd.va.gov/professional/newsletters/research-quarterly/v20n2.pdf

mydutytospeak. (2016, January 18). Soldier raped in Korea. https://mydutytospeak.com /2016/01/18/soldier-raped-in-korea/

Nassiri, J. M. (2017, January 6). 5 Things No One Tells You About Getting Out Of The Military. http://taskandpurpose.com/5-things-veterans-dont-know-getting-civilian-job

Rosenberg, M., & Philipps, D. (2015, December 3). All Combat Roles Now Open to Women, Defense Secretary Says. *The New York Times*. https://www.nytimes.com/2015/12/04/politics/combat-military-women-ash-carter.html

"Son, Men Don't Get Raped." http://www.gq.com //long-form/male-military-rape

The Fighter - The New York Times. https://www .nytimes.com/2016/12/28/magazine/afghanistan-soldier-ptsd-the-fighter.html?_r=2

To Rape is to Want Sex, Not Power | Quillette. http:// quillette.com/2016/01/02/to-rape-is-to-want-sex-not-power/

Chapter Three

The Long & Winding Road

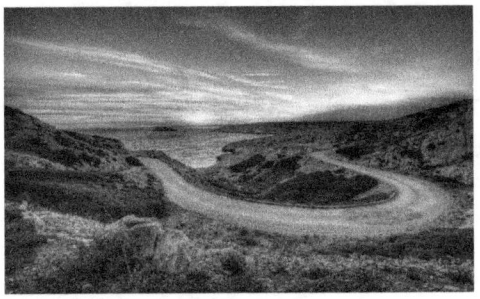

The meaning behind Paul McCartney's song *The Long and Winding Road* has been open to many interpretations; e.g. an unrequited love, the Beatles breakup, the unattainable, etc., but can also be a pretty darn good metaphor for life. Our personal journey will carry us along on some of the most delightful adventures but will most assuredly present us with struggles, challenging us to learn the lessons within the pain. It is the manner in which we embrace these struggles that not only defines who we are but who we will become.

https://paintyourlandscape.com/about/

I begin this chapter with an anecdote of a 20-year-old officer being told that: "You suffered a very serious injury and now you're broken." In my reading the story, I thought our Veteran may have experienced a panic attack. However, based on the information provided, I really didn't see the basis for diagnosing him with PTSD that resulted in a medical discharge. Can you imagine the effect that the few words coming out of that doctor's mouth had on his patient?

There's a number of points for me that come out of the story. I question how this officer transitioned back into civilian life? I wonder if he were ever able to get those words out of his mind? I'm also wondering how many more of our military that doctor wounded with his cutting words?

There are many ways a relatively straight path can be transformed into a winding and challenging quest. Now imagine that the Veteran you will be reading about is your loved one? How do you remove the scar but then, I'm guessing you would never be told about it.

****

. . . I wound up sitting in the psychiatrist's office. . . I told him everything I knew or could remember. . . about a recent situation . . . called the Helo Dunker. . . a simulation of a helicopter that actually crashes in a large, deep, indoor pool, and passengers have to try to make it out alive. During the night simulation, . . . I blacked out and nearly drowned before a scuba diver pulled me out.

I went on to explain that they were able to resuscitate me and I was also able to finish the training. . . I said to the doctor, So, what's the big deal? I walked out of there on my own. So I should be fine, right?

When I was done talking, he seemed to pause for a very long time before he said, 'Donald, have you heard of the term PTSD?' I nodded my head in a vague "yes." . . .He took his time . . . and then said, 'Donald, you don't seem to understand. You suffered a very serious injury and now you're broken.'

All the air seemed to go out of the room and I had difficulty breathing. I replied in a panic, 'What do you mean, I'm broken? . . . I need you to get me fixed up so I can make this deployment.' . . .

They're just going to have to find someone else," he said, ". . . We're going to help you get better, but it's going to take a long time and deployment for you just isn't an option anymore. I'm sorry.' ("People with Post

Traumatic Stress Disorder Heal with Story - viewcontent.cgi,")

****

A 2011 Pew Research Center article entitled "The Difficult Transition from Military to Civilian Life, written by Rich Morin, is an excellent resource. I strongly encourage you to read it in its entirety. I will highlight important aspects of this article as a preface to the direction I wish to take in this chapter.

"As you will learn, for many of our returning Veterans, the transition from military to civilian life is a relative straight and uncomplicated line. However, for close to 30% or more, this is not the case. A survey of 1,853 Veterans was conducted by The Pew Research Center who noted that:

"While more than seven-in-ten veterans (72%) report they had an easy time readjusting to civilian life, 27% say re-entry was difficult for them—a proportion that swells to 44% among veterans who served in the ten years since the Sept. 11, 2001, terrorist attacks.

". . . veterans who were commissioned officers and those who had graduated from college are more likely to have an easy time readjusting to their post-military life than enlisted personnel and . . . high school graduates.

". . . The lingering consequences of a psychological trauma are particularly striking: The probabilities of an easy re-entry drop from 82% for those who did not experience a traumatic event to 56% for those who did . . . In addition, those who served in a combat zone and those who knew someone who was killed or injured also faced steeper odds of an easy re-entry.

"Veterans who served in the post-9/11 period also report more difficulties returning to civilian life than those who served in Vietnam or the Korean War/World War II era, or in periods between major conflicts.

" Two other factors significantly shaped the re-entry experiences of post-9/11 veterans . . . Post-9/11 veterans who were married while they served had a significantly more difficult time readjusting than did married veterans of past eras or single people regardless of when they served.

"At the same time, higher levels of religious belief, as measured by frequent attendance at religious services, dramatically increases the odds that a post-9/11 veteran will have an easier time readjusting to civilian life." (Morin, 2011) I will explore some of these variables in detail also providing case stories where applicable beginning with an enlisted man's success story.

****

Brian Poole graduated high school on a Friday more than 21 years ago, and was on a bus to basic training for the U.S. Army in Fort Sill, Oklahoma, that Sunday. . . He saw combat in Afghanistan and Iraq, also served in Germany and South Korea, and was stationed at five bases in the U.S.

It was a challenging journey, which included two bronze stars from my time in combat zones," he says. In the Army, he says he learned that the definition of good leadership, and a strong team, is the same anywhere. "Traits like honor, integrity, and loyalty are universal."

While he was deployed, Brian completed several degrees with Army tuition assistance, and then later through the Post 9/11 GI bill, including an associate of arts in general studies; bachelors of science in theology and religion studies; a master of arts in psychology with a concentration in conflict resolution; and a graduate certificate in human resources management.

After he retired from the Army in 2013, he examined his experience and how he could apply it outside of the military. He realized his background in operations management, logistics, and human resources was applicable to the corporate world, and he started applying online for jobs. . .

For the past one-and-a-half years, Brian has worked in HR at Wells Fargo in Phoenix — overseeing personal, administrative, military, and Family Medical Leave Act leaves for team members. ("A veteran's advice on transition from military to civilian life," 2015)

****

I try to stay away from commenting too much on detailed scientific research in this book however, I found the following article, sent to me by a colleague, to be quite fascinating. The full article can be found in Science Daily, January 12, 2017.

To get to the point, researchers at Yale University have isolated the brain circuitry that coordinates predatory hunting in mice. They were able to isolate one set of neurons in the amygdala, the emotional center of emotion and motivation that cues the animal to pursue prey. "Another set signals the animal to use its jaw and neck muscles to bite and kill."

"The researchers used . . . light stimulation, to isolate and selectively activate each set of neurons. When the laser is off, the animals behave normally. But turn the laser on, and the mice take on qualities of "walkers" from The Walking Dead, pursuing and biting almost anything in their path, including bottle caps and wood sticks.

"We'd turn the laser on and they'd jump on an object, hold it with their paws and intensively bite it as if they were trying to capture and kill it," says lead investigator Ivan de Araujo, Associate Professor of Psychiatry at the Yale University School of Medicine and an Associate Fellow at the John B. Pierce Laboratory." ("Scientists switch on predatory kill instinct in mice,")

You might ask, what's the point here as mice are not men? Let's look into this interesting research a little further before I give you my interpretation of the findings. The author comments that:

"There must be some primordial subcortical pathway that connects sensory input to the movement of the jaw and the biting.

". . . By selectively manipulating the different types of neurons in this region, they found that one set of neurons controlled pursuit, and another controlled the kill. Experiments involved inanimate stand-ins for prey, such as sticks and bottle caps and animate bug-like toys, as well as live insects.

"The researchers also specifically lesioned each type of neuron. They found that, if they lesioned the neurons associated with biting and killing, the animals would pursue the prey but could not kill. The biting force of the jaw was decreased by 50 percent. "'They fail to deliver the killing bite,'" says de Araujo." (Han et al., 2017)

Now wouldn't it be wonderful if we could isolate this circuit among human being so there would be no more war. Okay, enough of the fanciful thinking so let's get real.

Our military is in the business of training our combat-ready troops to kill the enemy. However, they are not traditionally in the business of returning the wounded or emotionally troubled Veteran back to civilian life. Perhaps it's time to consider that as part of a transitional process. You've read earlier of an enlisted soldier's transition that went well. Here is one that's gone sour:

****

ROCK SPRINGS, WYO. — The only light in the vast Wyoming darkness came from the lit end of another 5:30 a.m. cigarette as Derric Winters waited alone for sunrise on the porch of his trailer. He never slept well, not anymore, so he smoked and stared across the three miles of barren landscape that separated him from town. He checked his voice mail, but there were no messages.

. . . His shirt read "ARMY," his hat read "10th Mountain Division," and his license plate read "Disabled Veteran." Five bullets rattled on his dashboard as he swerved around another car with his right fist pressed against the horn. "Come on," he said. "Go. Just go!"

It had been five years since he returned from 16 months at war, and some days he still acted like he was back in Afghanistan. Many days, he wished that he were.

What the hell am I supposed to do next. . . when he was medically discharged from the Army, which had provided his income, his sense of purpose, his self-esteem and 15 of his closest friends in a platoon they called "The Brotherhood."

He had tried to replace the war by working construction, roughnecking in the oil fields and enrolling in community college. He had tried divorce and remarriage; alcohol and drugs; biker gangs and street racing; therapy appointments and trips to a shooting range for what he called "recoil therapy." . . . Another day from killer to civilian," he continued. "Ugh. I miss it. ("'Ugh. I miss it.,'")

****

"A number of factors proved to be poor predictors of transition from military to civilian life including the following: ". . . race and ethnicity (separate variables tested the effect of being white, black, Hispanic or some other race); age at time of discharge; whether the veteran had children younger than 18 while serving; how long the veteran was in the military; and how many times the veteran had been deployed. (Morin, 2011)

Are those who return with the "Invisible Wounds" of war to experience the horrors of conflict each time they sleep or are triggered by an upsetting trigger. I believe that there is little issue that a preponderance of our returned Veterans with PTSD constitutes the bulk of those who have difficulty in the transition process.

There is also little debate that those with the condition tend to be only partially responsive to current therapies and psychotropic medication management. I personally consider the continuing symptoms of insomnia and nightmares after treatment to represent treatment failure. This measure is not universal but my own.

I will briefly review a few of the current frontline therapy interventions that are referred to as "Gold Standard Treatments." If you are interested in more detail, my 2nd book, *"Brain on Fire"* in Chapter Six – Emerging Therapies, goes into much greater depth than I provide in this book.

Now I must tell you that after my 47-years of clinical practice, I am absolutely and unashamedly biased. Please receive my perspective with a grain of salt. Even better, do your own inquiry through computer search about treatments for PTSD, only please do it through a skeptic's eyes. Perhaps your distrust of so-called front-line treatments will be further substantiated through the following 2015 study. The authors note that:

"Two trauma-focused therapies, cognitive processing therapy (CPT) and prolonged exposure, have been the most frequently studied psychotherapies for military-related PTSD. Five RCTs (Randomized Controlled Trials) of CPT (that included 481 patients) and 4 RCTs of prolonged exposure (that included 402 patients) met inclusion criteria.

". . . Forty-nine percent to 70% of participants receiving CPT and prolonged exposure attained clinically meaningful symptom improvement (defined as a 10- to 12-point decrease in interviewer-assessed or self-reported symptoms).

"However, mean post-treatment scores for CPT and prolonged exposure remained at or above clinical criteria for PTSD, and approximately two-thirds of patients receiving CPT or prolonged exposure retained their PTSD diagnosis after treatment (range, 60%-72%). CPT and prolonged exposure were marginally superior compared with non-trauma-focused psychotherapy comparison conditions.

"Conclusion: In military and veteran populations, trials of the first-line trauma-focused interventions CPT and prolonged exposure have shown clinically meaningful improvements for many patients with PTSD.

"However, nonresponse rates have been high, many patients continue to have symptoms, and trauma-focused interventions show marginally superior results compared with active control conditions. There is a need for improvement in existing PTSD treatments and for development and testing of novel evidence-based treatments, both trauma-focused and non-trauma-focused." (Steenkamp, Litz, Hoge, & Marmar, 2015)

You have read a well-respected review of the two primary "Gold Standard Treatments" I'll begin our discussion of these treatments with my least favorite intervention called Prolonged Exposure Therapy. Sounds scary, doesn't it? Interestingly, I use

Exposure Therapy in a novel way to end the nightmare of PTSD. You will learn more about this in another chapter of this book.

The proponents of Prolonged Exposure Therapy view this intervention as a proven way to lessen the power of memory, thoughts, and emotion related to trauma through a repetitious oral presentation of the trauma-related situations with a therapist. Prolonged Exposure Therapy is the most heavily studied PTSD treatment.

"The therapy generally consists of eight to fifteen sessions, with each session lasting approximately 60-90 minutes. The therapist using Prolonged Exposure works with the individual to promote emotional processing of traumatic memories through different types of exposure techniques.

"This therapy supports the idea that PTSD results from the individual's inability to process the memories surrounding the traumatic event because the individual intentionally avoids thoughts, emotions, and situations that are in some way connected to the traumatic event." ("A Systematic Review of Cognitive Processing Therapy and Prolonged Exposure with Veterans - viewcontent .cgi,")

Exposure therapy employs several methods to support the reduction of troubling emotional responses. Exposure therapists will conduct assessments to determine what combination of techniques will prove most effective.

Types of Exposure:

- **Imaginal Exposure:** In this type of exposure, a person in therapy is asked to mentally confront the fear or situation by picturing it in one's mind. For example, a person with . . . a fear of crowded places, might imagine standing in a crowded mall.

- **In Vivo Exposure:** When using this type of exposure, a person is exposed to real-life objects and scenarios. For example, a person with a fear of flying might go to the airport and watch a plane take off.

- **Virtual Reality Exposure:** This type of exposure combines elements of both imaginal and in vivo exposure so that a person is placed in situations that appear real but are actually fabricated. For example, someone who has a fear of heights . . .might participate in a virtual simulation of climbing down a fire escape.

Specific Exposure Therapy Techniques:

- **Systematic Desensitization:** This technique incorporates relaxation training, the development of an anxiety hierarchy, and gradual exposure to the feared item or situation. The relaxation training might include progressive muscle relaxation, soothing sights and sounds, and/o guided imagery. . . Then, during the gradual exposure to the ranked items, the learned relaxation techniques are applied to offset stress and anxiety.

- **Graded Exposure:** This technique is similar to systematic desensitization, but does not integrate the use of relaxation techniques.

- **Flooding:** In this technique, exposure can be in vivo or imaginal. A person is intensely exposed to anxiety-evoking events for a prolonged period of time. Flooding is usually done until the anxiety is significantly diminished.

- **Prolonged Exposure (PE):** Proven effective with trauma-related issues, this technique is similar to flooding but also incorporates psychoeducation and cognitive processing. ("Exposure Therapy,")

Researcher Alicia E. Meuret of the Department of Psychology at Southern Methodist University in

Texas wanted to examine Prolonged Exposure Therapy further. She assessed 34 individuals with panic/fear of being in large or unknown public places.

"She found that the participants all experienced increases in panic and anxiety during the sessions, as evidenced by physiological markers and emotional responses, but that these increases did not lead to better outcomes. In fact, the more panicked and fearful the individuals were, the worse their treatment outcomes.

"Additionally, in contrast to existing research, Meuret found that symptom reduction during treatment did not predict treatment outcome. In other words, even if the individuals experienced spikes in treatment severity during exposure and then were able to reduce their anxiety as the session continued, this drop did not lead to better overall outcome." ("Exposure Therapy for Anxiety Backfires in Study," 2012) An example of a negative outcome follows.

****

After briefly surveying my time in Iraq with a therapist, . . . I was asked to tell the story of my near-death experience in an IED ambush in Baghdad in 2007. In the sessions that followed, I retold this story dozens of times.

Whenever I tried to change the subject . . . I was told that the only way forward was to tell my IED ambush story over and over until it no longer bothered me or got my heart rate up. Repetition is the key, Scott explained.

After telling the story of my close call in Baghdad roughly 100 times, I began to have trouble sleeping. Eventually, I broke down altogether and was unable to read, write, or leave the house. One night after my cellphone failed to dial out, I stabbed it repeatedly with a stainless steel kitchen knife until I bent the blade 90 degrees. (Morris & Miller, 2015)

****

To stay fair and balanced, I will now provide you with a story that resulted in a positive outcome through PET. I earlier noted that I use Exposure Therapy as part of the RESET Therapy process. I want to activate the emotional circuitry in the brain in order to turn off the fear/anger/etc., switch. However, I tell my patients that you will only need to do this **one more time!**

****

With her eyes closed and a nervous smile, Tyhira Stovall wiggled uncomfortably . . . at her therapist's office in Philadelphia. As part of her treatment for post-traumatic stress disorder (PTSD) five years ago, (she) had been asked to revisit a terrifying experience.

. . . Slowly, she began to recount what happened to her more than a year before on the afternoon she skipped high school. . . As details started pouring out, the teen – with her eyes still shut – squirmed in the office chair, covered her face with her hands and rested her head against the wall, shaking with sobs.

. . . Stovall was an outgoing teenager before her rape. Afterwards, she described herself as a "walking zombie." She couldn't hug anybody, or look at her father, who she said had a similar look to her rapist. Her mother started homeschooling her, because she was too anxious to go to school. And she stopped dancing.

She lost her dance, she lost her joy. She just became like a shell," said her mother Juanita Sojourner. . . The therapy isn't easy . . . According to Capaldi, a clinical psychologist at the University of Pennsylvania, it often takes 14 to 17 sessions before a patient finds success.

Now, Stovall is preparing to graduate college and expecting her first child. She also started dancing again. "On stage, Stovall spins, wraps her arms around herself and then extends her leg high into the air. "In this moment, I claim myself as not being a victim," she said. "But I am a rape survivor. (8thday, 2014)

****

Cognitive Behavioral Therapy (CBT) is the next major intervention that claims to resolve the effects of trauma. I told you previously that I was biased. I'll lay it out there straight-forwardly in that I simply don't believe that the emotional center of the brain (where the cobra lives) responds to talk. Rather, when it comes to the power of emotion vs thought, I'd bet that emotion wins out nine times out of ten!

A blog by Stacey Freedenthal, PhD, LCSW explores the mechanisms thought to be central to CBT. She notes that:

"an event leads to thoughts, which lead to feelings – is the central premise of cognitive behavioral therapy (CBT). Thoughts also influence physiological reactions, behaviors, and further thoughts. In the CBT model, negative thoughts in themselves do not cause emotional problems, if those thoughts are realistic.

"There's the rub. Many of the things we tell ourselves simply are not true, or their truth is impossible to determine – thoughts like, 'I always screw up' or 'I'm a bad person' or 'I need to do everything right' or 'I'll never feel better.'

"Negative beliefs about oneself, others, or life can lead to (or exacerbate) many emotional problems, such as depression, anxiety, and even suicidal thoughts. So, the major goals of CBT are for people to learn to recognize their unhealthy thoughts, challenge them, change them, or observe them without believing and acting on them.

". . . One challenge is that you often are unaware of the thoughts that come before your moods and behaviors. Another challenge is that if you have strong negative thoughts about yourself, you have probably had these thoughts tens of thousands, perhaps even millions, of times in your life.

"You almost certainly treat these thoughts as facts. It takes a lot of practice to unlearn or otherwise disarm what you have regarded to be truths for many years." ("What is Cognitive Behavioral Therapy (CBT)?," 2013) When specifically focused towards our combat Veterans, CBT might be utilized in the following manner:

". . . therapists help patients understand that they are no longer caught in the traumatic situation, and give them tools to cope with negative thoughts and emotions. They work to un-train minds conditioned by the constant danger and uncertainty of combat.

 The instinct to always be armed can be life-saving in combat, but can interfere with civilian life. 'The idea in this cognitive therapy is to figure out what thinking is impeding recovery,' Monson said." ("Mis-Treating Our Veterans » Scienceline," 2007)

I must admit to you that I am a maverick. I don't like routine and I certainly rebel against providing therapy step by step according to a manual. Furthermore, applying these principles within a group setting is an absolute no-no in my mind.

I distinctly remember one of the Veterans I treated telling me that he had to get out of the group therapy room as quickly as his legs would take him because he was being triggered by another guy's story. With this in mind, try to imagine the gut reaction I have to the following description of CBT.

"Cognitive Processing Therapy is a 12 session evidence-based manualized treatment with a cognitive therapy focus and an optional written trauma account component . . . The therapy can be adapted for military trauma as well as group therapy.

". . . According to this treatment model, PTSD is thought to be an inability to recover from a traumatic event, and if an event is extremely severe, nearly everyone would have symptoms reflective of PTSD.

"The therapist begins by educating the participant on the symptoms of PTSD and the ways in which these symptoms may impact functioning and wellness. For example, the therapist may explain that individuals may feel safe and content when they feel emotionally numb, but this also leads to the inability to experience happiness and excitement.

"The therapist explains the way individuals form beliefs about themselves and the world, and how these beliefs are often altered after a traumatic event, which leads to negative generalizations or self-blame.

"The therapist asks the individual to write a brief impact statement explaining why the individual believes the event happened and to explain how the event has impacted life in regards to safety, trust, power and control, esteem, and intimacy.

"The therapist then works to identify stuck points in the impact statement which may be preventing the individual from processing the event, acknowledging emotions, and moving forward.

"The therapist educates the individual on emotions, and works with the patient to identify the connection between events, thoughts, emotions, and behavior. (and so on and so on)." ("A Systematic Review of Cognitive Processing Therapy and Prolonged Exposure with Veterans - viewcontent.cgi,") So once again, here's a success story to counterbalance my resistance to this routinized, utterly boring intervention.

****

Each time Andy Strunk stood up to give a work presentation, the same few doubts ran through his head. "Am I qualified to be in front of these people? Who am I? Why am I credible to be here?" worried Strunk, a 37-year-old marketing manager at a technology company in San Francisco.

But about a month ago, Strunk decided he had had enough. To progress in his career, he would need to tackle his public speaking fears now. "I don't want to have my life dictated by this thing that is anxiety," he says. So Strunk began seeing a psychologist, who is using a form of treatment called cognitive behavior therapy, or CBT, to help Strunk catch the negative thoughts before they begin – and replace them with the truth.

I've rewired my thinking to say, 'I am credible to be here,'" says Strunk, who mentally lists his accomplishments before taking the stage. . . For Strunk, the therapy is a welcome alternative to the anxiety-reducing and sleep-inducing pills his internist originally prescribed. "It feels like I'm a little bit more in control of things that would typically go unchecked in my head," he says. "That's what I was after. ("When Your Therapist Is a Computer ,.")

****

The final therapy I'd like to cover in this chapter is Eye Movement Desensitization Reprocessing (EMDR). The following clinic has actually taken a public position that they are no longer recommending this form of treatment. The authors note that:

EMDR is a treatment that was popular a couple of decades ago, but has fallen out of favor with evidence-based therapists in the past ten years. It is a treatment very similar to prolonged exposure, with the unusual addition of eye movement exercises paired with the exposure.

"All of the recent research on EMDR has shown that the eye movement adds nothing to the treatment, and thus clinicians more connected to up-to-date psychology practices have discontinued using it in favor of the more research-based prolonged exposure.

"It is not harmful, and many people in fact have benefitted from it. However, it is unclear why people persist in providing this antiquated treatment given what we now know about the active ingredients in therapy, other than not being familiar with the research about what works in therapy.

"Needless to say, we do not provide this treatment at Cognitive Behavioral Therapy Los Angeles, and we do not recommend it." ("What is Cognitive Behavioral Therapy (CBT)?," 2013)

I've provided you an overview (from my perspective of course) of the primary "Gold Star" interventions still utilized for the treatment of PTSD. Later in the book in my chapter, "The Sound That Heals," I will share with you a treatment that I truly believe can alter established trauma circuitry no matter how long it has gone on for.

I further hold that therapies that can change existing brain circuitry altered by trauma, address the issue through sensory as opposed to cognitive forms of intervention. The truth be told, there are still:

"More than half (56%) of all veterans who experienced a traumatic event say they have had flashbacks or repeated distressing memories of the experience, and nearly half (46%) say they have suffered from post-traumatic stress. Predictably, those who suffer from PTS were significantly less likely to say their re-entry was easy than those who did not (34% vs. 82%).

"According to the model, serving in a combat zone reduces the chances that a veteran will have an easier time readjusting to civilian life (78% for those who did not serve in a combat zone to slightly more than 71% for those who did).

Knowing someone who was killed or injured also lessens the probability that a veteran will have an easy re-entry by six percentage points (73% vs. 79%)." (Morin, 2011)

Summary

I've given you examples and numbers related to how a straight line for a successful transition from a life in the military to that of a civilian might occur. In essence, those who do not suffer from the invisible wounds of war (PTSD and TBI) might expect minimal difficulties in their adjustment process.

Alternatively, those who have served in combat zones, engaged in combat, been physically, sexually or emotionally injured within that context, will be inclined to have a difficult transition having to take, "that long and winding road." For a few of these, the road never seems to come to an end.

I've reviewed three front-line therapies through my biased eyes with two of them referred to as "Gold Standard". I've also provided you with 'fair-warning' about these treatments by referencing a highly respected meta-analysis of their efficacy.

I've teased you by alluding to a treatment that is able to quiet the hooded cobra noting that this is one of a number of interventions that turn off the switch in the emotional center of the brain. The next chapter will explore the intrusive nature of PTSD's effect on family life. This has come to be called Secondary PTSD.

References

A Systematic Review of Cognitive Processing Therapy and Prolonged Exposure with Veterans - viewcontent.cgi. http://sophia.

stkate.edu/cgi/viewcontent.cgi?article=1419&
context=msw_papers

A veteran's advice on transition from military to
civilian life. (2015, July 2). https://stories.
wf.com/a-veterans-advice-on-transition-from-
military-to-corporate-life/

Exposure Therapy. http://www.goodtherapy.org
/learn-about-therapy/types/exposure-therapy

Exposure Therapy for Anxiety Backfires in Study.
(2012, November 8). http://www.
goodtherapy.org/blog/exposure-therapy-for-
anxiety-backfires-in-study-1108123

Han, W., Tellez, L. A., Rangel, M. J., Motta, S. C.,
Zhang, X., Perez, I. O., … Araujo, I. E. de.
(2017). Integrated Control of Predatory
Hunting by the Central Nucleus of the
Amygdala. *Cell*, *168*(1), 311–324.e18.
https://doi.org/10.1016/j.cell.2016.12.027

Mis-Treating Our Veterans » Scienceline. (2007,
February 28). http://scienceline.org/2007/02
/policy_romero_ptsd/

Morin, R. (2011, December 8). The Difficult
Transition from Military to Civilian Life.
http://www.pewsocialtrends.org/2011/12/08/t
he-difficult-transition-from-military-to-
civilian-life/

Morris, D. J., & Miller, M. (2015, July 21). Trauma
Post Trauma. *Slate*. Retrieved from

http://www.slate.com/articles/health_and_scie
nce/medical_examiner/2015/07/prolonged_ex
posure_therapy_for_ptsd_the_va_s_treatment
_has_dangerous_side.html

People with Post Traumatic Stress Disorder Heal
with Story - viewcontent.cgi. http://
digitalcommons.georgefox.edu/cgi/viewconte
nt.cgi?article=1105&context=dmin

Scientists switch on predatory kill instinct in mice.
https://www.sciencedaily.com/releases/2017/
01/170112130133.htm

Slater, L. (2003, November 2). The Cruelest Cure.
The New York Times. http://www.nytimes.
com/2003/11/02/magazine/the-cruelest-
cure.html

"Ugh. I miss it." http://www.washington post.com
/sf/national/2014/04/19/ugh-i-miss-it/

What is Cognitive Behavioral Therapy (CBT)?
(2013, May 24). http://www.speaking
ofsuicide.com/2013/05/23/what-is-cbt/

When Your Therapist Is a Computer http://
health.usnews.com/health-news/health-
wellness/articles/2015/07/31/does-online-
cognitive-behavior-therapy-work

Chapter Four

Twists and Turns

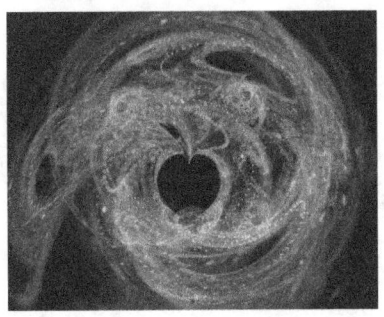

And when pain bites, men bargain. Boys too. We twist and turn, we plead and beg, we offer our tormentors what he wants so that the hurting will stop. And when there is no torturer to placate, no hooded man with hot irons and tongs, just a burn you can't escape, we bargain with God, or ourselves, depending on the size of our egos.

Mark Lawrence

I am sure that a number of those who experience a smooth transition free of twists and turns still carry within them the altered neuronal network created by their prior exposure to trauma. I discussed this matter in detail in my book entitled *PTSD Comorbid Conditions*. Since this was a book for professional therapists focused on PTSD, I will abbreviate the following material as I believe that it is important for you to be aware of some emerging material related to the aging of your Veteran.

Up to this point, I've discussed those who have served our country relatively recently. Unfortunately, it's not over that easily. I hold the perspective that PTSD, when untreated or improperly treated, affects the body and mind in a chronic, systemic and progressively destructive manner.

I bring to your awareness the gradual trickle of research that is supportive of my belief that PTSD is a systemic difficulty that, among other things, produces an inflammatory reaction in the brain. Findings related to the topic of aging Veterans and dementia is particularly startling to me in that it suggests that combat-incurred PTSD may lead to an early aging effect in our senior Veterans. If you are interested in where the research comes from in this discussion, please refer to my *PTSD Comorbid* book for these details in Chapter One, Dementia.

The second alarming finding suggests that combat veterans with PTSD are twice as likely as their non-combat colleagues to develop a dementing disorder as they age. Yet another study of those Veterans with sleep difficulties suggested that they are 27% more likely to develop dementia as compared to their colleagues without sleep disturbance.

When I discuss this topic with people the typical response is, "Wow, that's a lot of heavy stuff." I agree; indeed, it is but we're not done yet! About 10% of older Veterans are evidencing delayed-onset post-traumatic stress disorder (DOPTSD) among those Veterans who have served decades ago. This is like a time-bomb with a delayed fuse that our Veterans are carrying around inside of themselves. Now to be clear, these prior combat Veterans had shown no symptoms previously.

Now I personally find the above material to be staggering in its potential impact. To restate it differently, if the service member experienced combat involvement, he or she is likely to: physically age earlier; have a sleep disorder; be twice as likely to develop a dementing condition as compared to his/her service colleagues who did not engage in combat.

According to the National Health and Resilience in Veterans Study, the investigators found that over 60% of our Veterans are over 55 years of age.

If the referenced material is accurate, we need to begin planning immediately for the onslaught of those aging Veterans who will be filling our already pressed nursing homes for additional space. Alternatively, we might come to the conclusion that PTSD is indeed a systemic issue and invest in methodology to reset trauma circuitry in the brain back to its pre-trauma state. I now return to discuss some of the twists that the 2011 Pew Research Center investigated such as:

". . . The lingering consequences of a psychological trauma are particularly striking: The probabilities of an easy re-entry [into society] drop from 82% for those who did not experience a traumatic event to 56% for those who did . . . In addition, those who served in a combat zone and those who knew someone who was killed or injured also faced steeper odds of an easy re-entry. (Morin, 2011)

Many of the 56% referred to above attempt to deal with PTSD in ways readily and immediately available to them such as self-medication. It is quite logical for an afflicted person to do this in order to quiet, even for a while, the demons stirring within.

What those who choose this path don't realize is that this is a turn in the road that propels them down an ever-narrowing path leading to self-annihilation. I believe that it is crucial for family members to fully understand this destructive process.

While the title of this book specifically implies military personnel, I believe that the same eventual outcome is experienced by some of our First Responders as well as civilians who carry the scars of prior traumatic experiences. The author of the following webpage makes the connection between trauma and use of alcohol quite concisely noting that:

"During traumatic events the brain may partially shut down in order to prevent more extensive damage. Similar to a circuit breaker that is designed to protect multiple electrical outlets in a home from a sudden surge of electricity due to a lightning strike, the brain has a type of psychological shutdown that helps a person survive stressful situations.

"The problem is that unless those emotional circuits are reactivated and the pent-up emotions are processed thoroughly, they tend to stay in the person's brain in a sort of locked-down situation.

"It is extremely common for individuals struggling with PTSD to self-medicate with alcohol or other chemicals. When high levels of alcohol are consumed, the brain releases a naturally occurring chemical called dopamine. This washes over specialized receptors in the brain and relieves underlying psychological distress for a short time.

"The symptoms always return and too frequently they come back even stronger than they were before. The body develops a tolerance to alcohol very quickly. This means that the affected person will need larger and more frequent doses of alcohol in order to feel the desired effect.

"Between the brain's need for emotional relief and the individual's increasing tolerance to alcohol, addiction can develop very quickly. As many as 80 percent of alcoholics suffer from at least one underlying or co-occurring psychological disorder, such as PTSD or depression." ("How Alcohol Affects PTSD | Trauma Abuse Treatment,")

****

"Brian, a social drinker when he signed up for the Army nearly 12 years ago, said he began drinking in earnest after his first deployment to Iraq in 2003. Involved in four separate bomb attacks in that one tour, "I started drinking heavily to mask the pain." No one, he said, would have respect for a commander who whined about his pain and took sick leave. "Every night it was a minimum of a 12-pack, up to 24," he said. "I stayed at home, would sit and drink until 10 'o clock. I'd drink until my body shut down.

"By Brian's third tour in 2005, he was slamming the "near beers" you could buy on base that smelled like the real thing and had a very low alcohol content. He'd also get real beer in care packages from friends and family that didn't realize he was addicted.

"His soldiers would sometimes smell the alcohol on him, but Brian said he'd always have an excuse to brush it off. When a potential fourth tour raised questions about his physical ability to lead his command -- he'd had multiple shoulder surgeries and had mesh implanted in his abdomen -- Brian was put into the Army's Warrior Transition Unit for injured soldiers.

"And that's where he realized he had to stop drinking. He called his wife and told her he was going to get treatment. He later found out she'd already been planning to take the children and leave him." ("Army Alcoholics: More Soldiers Seeking Treatment for Alcohol Abuse - ABC News,")

****

Another twist along the self-medicating path is the Veteran's choice to use marijuana as an agent to deal with his condition. There is a movement in this country to make marijuana available for medicinal purposes in a number of states. I will provide you with the pros and cons in regards to this agent beginning with a reference to a 2016 webpage article in *Behavioral Pharmacology*. The author informs us that:

"Preliminary studies in humans also suggest that treatment with cannabinoids (marijuana) may decrease PTSD symptoms including sleep quality, frequency of nightmares, and hyperarousal. However, there are no large-scale, randomized, controlled studies investigat-ing this specifically.

"Studies in animal models have shown that cannabinoids can prevent the effects of stress on emotional function and memory processes, facilitate fear extinction, and have an anti-anxiety-like effect in a variety of tasks." ("Cannabinoids and post-traumatic stress disorder,")

The above description sounds wonderful so why aren't we using it preventively to stop the 20 Veterans who commit suicide daily? There are multiple factors involved in this matter, some of them legal, some of them moral, etc. I will try my utmost to give you a fair perspective of this drug, its benefits and its drawbacks.

I said before that I'd try not to be too technical in this book for families. However, I couldn't avoid sharing the 'kill switch' article with you in an earlier chapter. I'm going to break my rule again by discussing the findings of an Israeli chemist, Dr. Raphael Mechoulam, who identified THC as the psychoactive compound in marijuana.

He began his research in the early 60's by securing marijuana through breaking the law. He got away with it because the supplier happened to be the police. Since chemists' in general tend to be technical, I'll try to translate where I can for the purpose of your better understanding.

"In 1988, Dr. Allyn Howett uncovered the binding sites for THC in the human brain which were found to be in the hippocampus, frontal cortex and the cerebellum referencing these sites as 'cannabinoid.' As an aside, many of these sites are similar to the sites that become hyper-aroused in those with PTSD.

"Another aspect of THC is that its derivatives help to maintain balance (homeostasis) in the body. Here's where D. Mechoulam gets somewhat technical: "As smoothly as keys fit into a lock, THC binds to cannabinoid receptor and ignites a series of chemical reactions. This causes changes in your brain and body.

"When THC engages the brain, you'll experience altered behavioural and cognitive ability. These changes aren't necessarily negative changes unless you find them uncomfortable. Mostly, THC will just make you feel different than you normally do. Once you get used to how it feels to consume THC, you'll find that you can perform all of your normal daily activities just fine. "In a way, THC is similar to trying on a new pair of glasses. It causes you to see and experience things in a different way.

"Cognitive and behavioral changes are not the only effects of THC, however. The cannabinoid engages the immune system, quelling inflammation. It spurs appetite, triggering the release of hunger hormones and jump-starting your metabolism. It can also have a sedative effect, making you feel blissful and sleepy." ("THC: Everything You Need To Know About Delta9-Tetrahydrocannabinol,")

My interpretation of this phenomena is that it is a temporary switch effect that approximates the neuronal circuit's previously balanced state. Now this may sound like pretty good news to our Veterans and indeed, many of them are moving to take this bend in the road. I'm providing you with an example of someone choosing this path.

****

Roberto Pickering's story is all too familiar. The infantry Marine says he fought during the invasion of Iraq in 2003, lost some 'good buddies' and returned to civilian life a 'basket case' from battling a new enemy: post-traumatic stress disorder. Pickering says he was pumped full of medications — from Valium to Zoloft, OxyContin, Seroquel, Lithium, Ambien and more — by Department of Veterans Affairs doctors.

He tried to go back to school but had trouble adjusting. He recoiled further after one friend took his own life and another died of a heroin overdose after becoming dependent on opioids through his medical care. Pickering moved into his parents' California basement and found solace in the bottle while his life spiraled out of control.

Unlike thousands of post-9/11 veterans who have committed suicide, Pickering then found another way to cope: He began experimenting with marijuana about 10 years ago. 'This war doesn't end when you come back,' he said. Cannabis "really improved my quality of life … I found what works for me.

Using marijuana regularly, he said, his angry outbursts diminished and he was able to get a good night's sleep. He said he was able to kick his drinking habit and, best of all, he didn't have to take the litany of pills he calls toxic.

Pickering said he usually smokes a bit at night and calls himself a responsible family man, far from the stereotype of a coach-potato stoner. He doesn't know why marijuana changed his life, and researchers can only guess, because the plant has never been studied as a treatment for veterans' PTSD. Despite state ballot initiatives to legalize marijuana for medical and nonmedical use in recent years, earlier this month it again received the highest drug classification by the Drug Enforcement Administration." ("Study,")

****

Let's take a look at some of the negative side effects that one might expect from the prolonged use of marijuana. Someone suffering from PTSD isn't necessarily going to ponder long-term effects particularly when some relief is gained. In this context, family members are in a better position to have this awareness so here goes:

- **Alterations in memory:** One study has shown that heavy cannabis users have decreased verbal memory over time.

- **Bronchitis-like symptoms:** This is not from THC, but from smoking. If you smoke a lot for a long period of time, you may experience some lung irritation.

- **Tolerance:** When you consume a lot of THC regularly for long periods of time, your body develops a tolerance to the compound. This makes the herb less effective, and you'll have to consume more and more of it to see results.

- **Apathy:** This is related to tolerance. If you use cannabis excessively over long periods of time, your body stops being completely responsive to the herb. This can cause you to feel a little blank or emotionally numb.

- **Trouble for those with psychotic disorders:** If you are predisposed to a psychotic disorder, you might want to reconsider THC. Research has found that folks with a genetic vulnerability for schizophrenia and psychosis can develop symptom onset earlier when they regularly consume THC". ("THC: Everything You Need To Know About Delta9-Tetrahydrocannabinol,")

I've given you the pros and cons in regards to the use of marijuana to counter the symptoms of PTSD. The word counter is critical here in that the user must continue or the symptoms will represent. In other words, we have an underlying systemic disorder that has not been remediated but rather, has been medicated. Stop the drug, the effects come back.

What if we had an intervention that could turn off the symptoms, resetting the system back to normative functions? Would your Veteran choose this path or continue to choose marijuana because of its soothing qualities? Time will provide us with this answer as the means to reset brain circuitry becomes widely available and easy to access.

The third component of the chemical triangle is the use of legally prescribed medication to manage the symptoms of PTSD. Have you ever wondered how some drugs come to be legalized while others are not? For example, LSD is making a re-emergence with some who are seeking to legalize research among our Veterans with PTSD.

****

When former U.S. Army Specialist Kyle Wesolowski returned from Iraq in December 2010 following a brutal yearlong deployment, psychiatrists at the Fort Hood army post in Texas gave him "a cocktail of seven different drugs" for his anxiety, depression and other war-related mental health issues. .More than three years later, Wesolowski has come to an uncomfortable conclusion about the unintended consequences of ingesting those medications: They made him homicidal.

While desperately struggling to taper off the drugs without an exit strategy from his military doctors, Wesolowski contemplated murdering a young woman he met in a bar near the base.

When she talked to me, I put on a fake smile and tried to be nice," Wesolowski said, though in reality he recalled hating her for being happy and carefree, and now says that due to the side effects of his drug cocktail, he felt violent urges.

I began to fantasize about killing her," he said. ("'Medicating Our Troops Into Oblivion': Prescription Drugs Said To Be Endangering U.S. Soldiers,")

✶✶✶✶✶✶✶✶✶✶✶✶✶✶✶✶✶✶✶✶✶✶✶

"The violent tendencies of some mentally traumatized soldiers and veterans cannot be written off as an aberration," said Dr. Peter Breggin, a psychiatrist and author who's written extensively about the potential dangers of the use of psychotropic drugs to treat mental illness among servicemen and servicewomen.

"Breggin contends such episodes are the result of what he describes as a "massive prescription drug epidemic" that encompasses the Department of Defense and the Department of Veterans Affairs, in which tens of thousands of soldiers and veterans returning from traumatic tours of duty ingest drugs – in some cases multiple varieties – that can have significant side effects, including intensifying feelings of rage." ("'Medicating Our Troops Into Oblivion': Prescription Drugs Said To Be Endangering U.S. Soldiers,")

A rather scathing attack was published in Scientific American in 2013 by Kali Tal entitled, "PTSD: The Futile Search for the 'Quick Fix.'" The author states that:

"Military and pharmaceutical interests converge: the former wants quick or easy fixes, and the latter wastes no time in peddling the pharmaceutical flavor of the month, whether it's sertraline, paroxetine, fluoxetine, venlafaxine, risperidone, clonidine, diazepam, lorazepam, alpralozam, duloxetine, propranolol, prazosin, yohimbine, cortisol, quetiapine or gabapentin.

"In 2012, 'the Pentagon spent more on pills, injections and vaccines_than it did on Black Hawk helicopters, Abrams tanks, Hercules C-130 cargo planes and Patriot missiles—combined'; drug sales to the military doubled between 2001-2011. The military's hope is that a combination of drugs and short-term TFT will prove more effective than either alone.

"Between 2001-2011, the Defense and the VA combined spent $791 million on Risperidone, a drug that turned out to be no more effective than placebo for treating PTSD. Just last year, the Army finally changed its long-standing policy of prescribing benzodiazepines for soldiers with PTSD because the drugs are highly addictive, and they worsen PTSD symptoms." (Tal,)

Finally, while there are many illicit or formerly illicit drugs being used to attempt to control or alter PTSD symptoms, I'll discuss the big three: Ecstasy, LSD and the Magic Mushroom.

****

James . . ., a veteran combat medic who served in Afghanistan, and a freshman at the University of Colorado, told the student-run news . . . about his experience with MDMA-assisted therapy. He had tried every treatment the Department of Defense sponsors for PTSD — he took pills, went to therapy, and even bought a puppy — but saw little improvement.

Eventually he enrolled in a study in Boulder sponsored by MAPS, which looked at the efficacy of MDMA (Ecstasy) to treat PTSD. . . 'A good way to describe it is that I felt like I was in a cave, trying to get out, but I didn't have any light'" he said. 'So I was just feeling around the walls, getting turned around, and getting even more lost.'

But with the MDMA sessions, it was like the therapist was my guide and the MDMA was a flashlight. With those resources, I could get out of the cave I'd been lost in for so long.

...It blew me away, how effective it was...It gave me my life back. It was like a burden being lifted off my back for the first time in years. I could feel. I could love. It helped me more than I can even put into words. ("Soldier Uses Psilocybin To Treat PTSD,")

****

"I'm cautious but hopeful," said Dr. Charles R. Marmar, the head of psychiatry at New York University's Langone School of Medicine, a leading PTSD researcher who was not involved in the study.

'If they can keep getting good results, it will be of great use. PTSD can be very hard to treat. Our best therapies right now don't help 30 to 40 percent of people. So we need more options."

But he expressed concern about the potential for abuse. "It's a feel-good drug, and we know people are prone to abuse it," he said. "Prolonged use (Ecstasy) can lead to serious damage to the brain." (Philipps, 2016)

Let's take a look at some of that potential damage one week following use of MMDA. This material is forthcoming from the National Institutes of Health (NIH), National Institute of Drug Abuse, Advancing Addiction Science: MDMA (Ecstasy) Abuse.

"Reported Undesirable Effects (up to 1 week post-MMDA, or longer):
8. Anxiety
9. Restlessness
10. Irritability
11. Sadness
12. Impulsiveness
13. Aggression
14. Sleep Disturbances
15. Lack of appetite
16. Thirst
17. Reduced interest in and pleasure from sex
18. Significant reductions in mental abilities

Potential Adverse Health Effects:

- Nausea
- Chills
- Sweating
- Involuntary jaw clenching and teeth grinding
- Muscle cramping
- Blurred vision
- Marked rise in body temperature – (hyperthermia)
- Dehydration
- High Blood Pressure
- Heart failure
- Kidney failure
- Arrhythmia

Symptoms of MDMA Overdose:
- High Blood Pressure
- Faintness
- Panic attacks
- Loss of consciousness
- Seizures (Abuse,)

That's a pretty heavy adverse reaction list. Knowing about it, I'd be inclined to go for a non-invasive procedure with no known, long-lasting side effects if only that type of choice were available. But by now, my hints should be giving you the idea that such an intervention exists. Indeed, it does and it's called RESET Therapy.

Next, we're going back to the 60's to talk about the LSD thing. If you grandpas and grandmas were around during the Hippie era, they may have tried it themselves. It's like that old expression: what goes around comes around.

"It's been half a century since LSD was a thing, first extolled by some for 'opening' the mind, then excoriated by some for making some people jump out of windows to escape the giant pink cockroaches. Yet according to an analysis published in the Canadian Medical Association Journal, there are studies being done on use of lysergic acid diethylamide as a treatment for post-traumatic stress disorder, of all things. And anxiety.

". . . Now, decades later, the sensationalism has waned, research done in the 1950s and 1960s that had been quietly shelved is coming back to light, and it's in again to evaluate other effects the drugs have.

"'Keep in mind that it's different in many ways than what we may see in an abuse setting – when people came to the ER experiencing negative effects of these compounds,' says Dr. Matthew Johnson, associate professor of Psychiatry and Behavioral Sciences at the Johns Hopkins University School of Medicine, in a video interview.

"These drugs had a history, points out Johnson. Because of the bad name LSD and its ilk developed due to abuse, intriguing medical work with them got shelved." ("LSD staging comeback – to treat PTSD - Science & Medicine - Haaretz.com,")

Let's also look at the negative side effects that one could experience from using LSD and other hallucinogens.

Short-Term Effects
- Increased heart rate
- Increased blood pressure
- Heart failure
- Abnormal, rapid breathing
- Lung failure
- Changed emotional feelings
- Confusion
- Disorientation
- Suspiciousness
- Mixed-up speech
- Loss of muscle control
- Meaningless movements
- Irrational actions
- Violent behavior
- Distorted reality
- Aggressiveness
- Distorted sense of time and space
- Sense of relaxation and well-being
- Nausea and loss of appetite
- Chills and flushing
- Shaking
- Poor coordination
- Distorted body image, feeling of floating or out-of-body experiences
- Dilated eyes
- Seeing things that aren't really there
- Unpredictable trips, which can be pleasant or a nightmare, causing panic

Long-Term Effects
- Flashbacks weeks, months, or even years after the drug use
- Flashbacks may be set off by using other drugs or by physical exercise
- Flashbacks may be pleasant or a living nightmare
- Most flashbacks last a very short time, only a minute or two
- Decreased motivation
- Prolonged depression
- Increased panic
- Impaired memory and concentration
- Possible severe mental disturbances
- Psychosis
- Increased delusions
- Bad trips may last hours, weeks, and even months ("Short and Long Term Effects | Teens | Survive - Stop Yourself. Stop a Friend.,")

The following author reiterates many of the principles I include in my understanding of RESET Therapy regarding its underlying principles. This is one of those technical references I'm including but, be reassured that I will clarify it later in this chapter.

". . . research has shown, sights, sounds, scents and sensations from our sensory organs enter a region at the center of the brain called the thalamus. . . The processed material — sorted for context and assessed for significance . . . is returned to the thalamus, which then deposits it into the hippocampus, where it is stored as memory.

". . . The sensory memory of the trauma — which is still entangled with the emotion associated with that moment — passes through the thalamus and is stored directly in the hippocampus without processing in the more sophisticated parts of the brain.

"These raw memories, still tied to the fear response they provoked, are a constant threat to bolt into awareness as flashbacks, nightmares, hypervigilance or rage, which can trigger the fight-or-flight reflex centered in the amygdala.

". . . the repressive amygdala is overactive in people with PTSD, while the rationalizing power of the higher brain is suppressed. . . the opposite is true for someone given MDMA; the drug stimulates the prefrontal cortex and suppresses the amygdala. . . One of the drug's signature effects is a dramatic reduction in fear, a sense of 'being protected,' coupled with a rapid-fire run of novel insights.

"Passie theorizes that as the amygdala lets down its guard under the drug's quieting influence, the traumatic memories can reemerge from the hippocampus to be sent up for the higher processing the brain didn't do in the immediacy of the trauma.

". . . Now, at last, the conditions exist in the brain that allow traumatic memories to be properly contextualized . . ." ("Can psychedelic trips cure PTSD and other maladies? - The Washington Post,")

Since we're on a 'Magical Mystery Tour' (for you young folk, this is an album and television film the Beatles devised, wrote and directed which was broadcast on BBC Television at Christmas, 1967), recall that Paul McCartney noted:

"Because those were psychedelic times it had to become a magical mystery tour, a little bit more surreal than the real ones to give us a license to do it. But it employs all the circus and fairground barkers, 'Roll up! Roll up!', which was also a reference to rolling up a joint.

"We were always sticking those little things in that we knew our friends would get; veiled references to drugs and to trips. 'Magical Mystery Tour is waiting to take you *away*,' so that's a kind of drug, 'it's *dying* to take you away' so that's a Tibetan Book of the Dead reference.

"We put all these words in and if you were just an ordinary person, it's a nice bus that's waiting to take you away, but if you're tripping, it's dying, it's the real tour, the real magical mystery tour. We stuck all that stuff in for our 'in group' of friends really.

"Magical Mystery Tour was the equivalent of a drug trip and we made the film based on that. 'That'll be good, a far-out mystery tour. Nobody quite knows where they're going. We can take 'em anywhere we want, man!' Which was the feeling of the period.

"'They can go in the sky. It can take off!' In fact, in the early script, which was just a few fireside chats more than a script, the bus was going to actually take off and fly up the magicians in the clouds, which was us all dressed in red magicians' costumes, and we'd mess around in a little laboratory being silly for a while." ("Magical Mystery Tour | The Beatles Bible,")

Wow, after revisiting this time again, I'm inspired to discuss 'shrooms' a bit. The authors of the following study found that:

". . . low doses of the active ingredient in magic mushrooms repairs brain damage caused by extreme trauma, offering renewed hope to millions of sufferers of PTSD . . . The study confirms previous research by Imperial College London, that psilocybin, a naturally occurring compound present in "shrooms", stimulates new brain cell growth and erases frightening memories.

"Mice conditioned to fear electric shock when hearing a noise associated with the shock 'simply lost their fear', says Dr. Juan Sanchez-Ramos, who co-authored the study. A low dose of psilocybin led them to overcome 'fear conditioning' and the freeze response associated with it

". . . In the South Florida University study, the mice treated with low doses of psilocybin grew healthy new brain cells and their overactive medial prefrontal cortex regions (common in PTSD sufferers) were restored to normal functionality.

". . . Dr. Sanchez-Ramos acknowledged that there was no way of knowing whether the mice in the experiment experienced altered states of consciousness or hallucinations - commonly experienced with magic mushrooms, but he believed the doses were too low to cause psychoactive effects.

". . . Magic mushrooms could help millions recover from the debilitating cycles of fight and flight and other conditioned biological responses caused by extreme trauma, if only they weren't listed as a dangerous Schedule 1 drug with no medical benefits. ("Can psychedelic trips cure PTSD and other maladies? - The Washington Post,")

****

I realized what trauma could do to a person after coming home from each one of my three deployments. . . One day, three years after my first deployment, I remember waking up and asking myself: Who am I? What have I become? How was I not aware of this massive transformation?

I acquired a single . . . mushroom at a music festival, which probably weighed a gram and a half. I asked my best friend (also a veteran) if he wanted to sit with me while I went through the experience.

. . . This event has turned out to be one of the most significant, personal, and transformative events of my life. It trumped the firefights, the arguments, the let downs, the chronic stress. I remember feeling as though I was previously blind and seeing for the first time.

The beauty of life around me nearly brought me to tears. I was so reflective on my life but could only see the good. I had to struggle to think of anything unpleasant. Until that point I had never felt so lucky and blessed to be alive.

I saw my erratic and callous behavior with compassion and sympathy rather than resentment. I saw that I was running towards a cliff face and wanted to do a 180-degree turn. I saw what I had, and not what I lost. I remember thinking my innocence is not gone but only buried, and at that moment I decided that I wanted to dig it back up. . ." ("Personal Story,")

****

We'll end this exploration with a comment related to the potential short-term and long-term effects of this hallucinogenic agent.

Short-Term Effects
- Increased heart rate
- Increased blood pressure
- Heart failure
- Abnormal, rapid breathing
- Lung failure
- Changed emotional feelings
- Confusion
- Disorientation
- Suspiciousness
- Mixed-up speech
- Loss of muscle control
- Meaningless movements
- Irrational actions
- Violent behavior
- Distorted reality
- Aggressiveness
- Distorted sense of time and space
- Sense of relaxation and well-being
- Nausea and loss of appetite

- Chills and flushing
- Shaking
- Poor coordination
- Distorted body image, feeling of floating or out-of-body experiences
- Dilated eyes
- Seeing things that aren't really there
- Unpredictable trips, which can be pleasant or a nightmare, causing panic

Long-Term Effects
- Flashbacks weeks, months, or even years after the drug use
- Flashbacks may be set off by using other drugs or by physical exercise
- Flashbacks may be pleasant or a living nightmare
- Most flashbacks last a very short time, only a minute or two
- Decreased motivation
- Prolonged depression
- Increased panic
- Impaired memory and concentration
- Possible severe mental disturbances
- Psychosis
- Increased delusions
- Bad trips may last hours, weeks, and even months ("Short and Long Term Effects | Teens | Survive - Stop Yourself. Stop a Friend.,")

To wrap up this discussion, I'd like to briefly discuss another intervention that appears to engage the hyperactivated and hyper-aroused aspects of the neuronal network of PTSD. This procedure doesn't utilize a cocktail mix of medications or any single medication or drug. It is non-invasive and has no long-lasting side effects.

It is designed to modify the restoration of traumatic memories in the brain's circuitry. It doesn't seem to change the memory itself, in fact, after the interventions, the memory appears to be more complete and intact. What drops out is the emotional component that causes the discomfort.

There is no talk involved in this procedure other than the therapist guiding the patient to 'light up' the trauma experience(s) through the senses as though the event were unfolding for the first time. However terrifying it is, the patient is promised that he/she will only have to 'go through this one more time.'

Following the procedure, other than in Complex PTSD cases, the patient's trauma altered neuronal network changes from a defensive/protective function to its prior function of curiously/growth. The results are permanent.

This is the point where I try to make sense of all the stuff you've read about in this chapter. We'll start with the song from Sesame Street:

One of these things is not like the others,
One of these things just doesn't belong,
Can you tell which thing is not like the others
By the time I finish my song?

Did you guess which thing was not like the
others? Did you guess which thing just doesn't
belong? (Songwriters Joe Raposo and Jon
Stone)

Summary

I began this chapter with some astonishing facts
emerging from recent research regarding PTSD and
our aging veterans. The reason I did this was to bring
to your attention the fact that that trauma effects alter
the circuitry of the brain and simply don't disappear.
The combat Veteran who successfully and rapidly
completed the transition process, may find that in
his/her 60's, 70's and so on, the symptoms of PTSD
come roaring back.

This has been referred to as Delayed Onset Post-
Traumatic Stress Disorder. It is thought that the prefrontal lobes of the brain have kept this material from
surfacing. In some, when this area weakened due to
the aging process, lo and behold, the evil Genie is let
out of the bottle.

I've discussed my belief that sleep disorder,
insomnia, flashbacks and nightmares following

treatment represent 'a failed treatment.' I've also suggested that PTSD is akin to a brain wiring default that becomes frozen in an un-natural state. Over the decades, a price is exacted from a system that remains in a hyper-alert state. We are simply not designed to perpetuate the fight, flight or freeze stress response.

I wandered along divergent paths your loved one might take, whether they be in liquid, pill or 'shroom' forms. I slyly introduced a relatively new, neuro-scientific approach that addresses the cause of the difficulties rather than the symptoms.

I've tried to take a balanced position in all of this even though I informed you that I'm clearly biased. In the next chapter, I will take you through a discussion of the effects that PTSD has on family systems including the marriage, the children, divorce, and homelessness.

References

Army Alcoholics: More Soldiers Seeking Treatment for Alcohol Abuse - ABC News. http://abcnews.go.com/Health/army-alcoholics-soldiers-seek-treatment-alcohol-abuse/story?id=9863321

Can psychedelic trips cure PTSD and other maladies? - The Washington Post. https://

www.washingtonpost.com/national/health-science/can-acid-trips-cure-ptsd-and-other-maladies/2014/11/17/3eaeb59a-5ded-11e4-8b9e-2ccdac31a031_story.html?utm_term=.31c1cfe45ca7

Cannabinoids and post-traumatic stress disorder: clinical a... : Behavioural Pharmacology. http://journals.lww.com/behaviouralpharm/Fulltext/2016/10000/Cannabinoids_and_post_traumatic_stress_disorder__.1.aspx

How Alcohol Affects PTSD | Trauma Abuse Treatment. http://traumaabuse treatment .com/how-alcohol-affects-ptsd

LSD staging comeback – to treat PTSD - Science & Medicine - Haaretz.com. http://www .haaretz.com/israel-news/science/1.675115

"Medicating Our Troops Into Oblivion": Prescription Drugs Said To Be Endangering U.S. Soldiers. http://www.ibtimes.com /medicating-our-troops-oblivion-prescription -drugs-said-be-endangering-us-soldiers-1572217

Short and Long Term Effects | Teens | Survive - Stop Yourself. Stop a Friend. http://www2 .courtinfo.ca.gov/stopteendui/teens/resources/ substances/hallucinogens/short-and-long-term-effects.cfm#content

Soldier Uses Psilocybin To Treat PTSD. http:// reset.me/personal-story/soldier-uses-psilocybin-to-treat-ptsd/

Study: Can marijuana improve PTSD symptoms for veterans? https://www.stripes.com /news /study-can-marijuana-improve-ptsd-symptoms-for-veterans-1.427271

Chapter Five

Unraveling

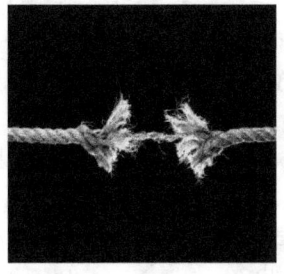

"I knew this for a fact.
Little by little,
the ache to see him, to hear him
would disappear.
Little by little I'd forget how his arms felt,
how his fingers felt, how his lips felt.
the sound of his voice, the intensity of his gaze, all
of it.
Trace by trace it would slip from my mind, recede
into foggy memory.
The painful haze that dulled my present
would melt into the past. Maybe not all the way,
maybe there would be a few scars.
Maybe I'd be different, but I'd be me again. Little
by little."

Jennifer DeLucy

In my earlier years, I received training from an eminent teacher, Dr. Salvador Minuchin, in an intervention referred to as Structured Family Therapy. As part of the training, I learned to 'join' with the family in order to learn their rules of non-verbal communication conveyed through behavioral interaction among varied family members.

I explored the subsets in the family such as the grandparents and how they supported or undermined the primary caretakers (parents). I watched and saw how they may have subtly supported the Identified Patient (IP) in the adolescent's rebellion against the parents. I might have also observed how one parent interacted with the other in addressing the primary issue.

Dr. Minuchin proposed that pathology in the family exists not in the individual but within the family system itself. I held this belief and practiced accordingly for many years. I would push for change by aligning with the excluded parent through fostering empowerment or, perhaps by having the grandparent cede power to the single parent rather than undermining her, etc.

My model of a healthy family unit was that of the presence of clear boundaries between generations. Did the parents function as an executive team consulting with each other as needed? Did the older siblings have more privileges that the younger ones? Were the older ones staying up later than the others? Did the family eat together?

Now add a couple of decades and I've modified my perspective particularly in regards to military families, especially when one comes home with PTSD. When the poison comes home with the Veteran, everyone in the family is exposed to it and becomes a potential victim to it.

Because of the importance of the family unit, this chapter will focus primarily on the agents of family stability, the parents. The following chapter will pick up on the offspring within the family, the children.

Some spouses or significant others, (here-after referred to as the spouse) simply can't handle it and the family/relationship breaks up, disintegrates and the couple move on with their separate lives. For those who choose to remain, they do this at a price, the sacrifice of their own spontaneity. Ultimately, they come to live in a world of fear and defensiveness. This reaction eventually comes to be called, "Secondary PTSD."

From my perspective, there's nothing secondary about it! If it walks like a duck, quacks and waddles like a duck, by God, it's a duck. Perhaps it's called 'Secondary' to avoid health insurers from having to pay to treat it. From my perspective, this is a rather condescending term suggesting a 'mini-me' version of PTSD that is both patronizing and offensive.

In my mind, all family members who have struggled in this tainted environment require detoxification.

Resetting the stability and viability of the couple is secondary only to normalizing the trauma circuitry in the brain of the primarily afflicted military member.

Unfortunately, the children in the family must wait until the prior two objectives are accomplished. It is at this point they enter the picture with a stabilized executive structure in place once again, that is designed to nourish and protect them. The following synopsis provides you with a brief example of the 'toxic' environment that emerges foremost in the spouse through initial exposure to PTSD:

"The signs, symptoms, and effects of Secondary PTSD in the spouse are just as varied as the ones exhibited by Veterans with 'primary' PTSD. . . Basically, when you're living with a veteran who has Post Traumatic Stress Disorder, you become his (or her) caretaker. You slip into a role, without even noticing it, that has you constantly watching for people or circumstances that might 'set him off.'

"You're trying to make sure everything stays in line - that nothing aggravates or upsets your vet – that everything is 'perfect.' Despite your best efforts, you're still getting screamed at and berated by the person you're trying to help on a much too frequent basis.

"Your vet is not emotionally 'there' for you. When you're upset or happy, angry or sad, you have to deal with your emotions on your own. You begin to feel ignored and unloved and start 'protecting' yourself by treating others - especially your vet - the same way.

"This cycle takes its toll on many spouses. You lose yourself. It's impossible to tiptoe around your vet, day in and day out, while taking care of all of life's other duties (duties normally shared between two people), without feeling the strain. And that strain soon transforms into... ta da...**Secondary PTSD**.

"Secondary PTSD may make you feel overly angry, depressed, exhausted (but, alas, unable to sleep), overwhelmed, and just plain unhappy with the world around you. I can honestly say there have been times when I found the idea of folding a load of laundry absolutely impossible.

"I felt like I could not do anything right. I cried a lot and was really, REALLY pissed at the world." (Street, NW, Washington, & Inquiries, 2011)

****

For the past 29 years, Darlene has lived with Bob, a Vietnam veteran diagnosed with PTSD. She describes this time as "walking on eggshells, never knowing when he'll blow." Over the years, to deal with her husband's reactivity, Darlene has increased her own vigilance. . . Many times she had to leave public gatherings due to her husband's confrontations.

As their marriage progressed, Darlene's continual vigilance took its toll, leaving her with many of the same symptoms as her husband. Her anticipation of 'a blowup at any moment' created distance in her relationships – not only with family members, but also with friends. She complains that she has had no social life. ("Secondary PTSD,")

****

An investigative team eloquently suggested that trauma has the capacity to resonate throughout the family system, pulling others into its destructive influence. . . The authors' note:

"Psychic trauma may be likened to a stone thrown into a pool of water. It creates ripples that affect not only the victims themselves, but also those who are close to them. The term secondary traumatization . . . has been used to indicate that others who come into close contact with a trauma victim may experience considerable emotional upset and may, over time, themselves become indirect victims of the trauma.

"Detrimental effects of trauma on significant others have been observed among spouses and children of both Vietnam veterans . . . and Holocaust survivors . . . as well as in therapists of trauma victims. Yet, while extensive study has systematically documented both immediate and delayed disorders among primary trauma victims . . . most of the evidence for the impact of trauma on family members stems from clinical observations based on small and unrepresentative samples.

".. . This study attempts to begin to fill in the gap by exploring the impact of psychic trauma among combat veterans on the mental and physical health of those who are closest to them, their wives. . . The marital relationship appears to be particularly vulnerable to problems stemming from the veterans' traumatic combat experiences. Studies of Vietnam combat veterans have found a significantly higher incidence of dyadic maladjustment.

".. . wives who reported current PTSD symptoms in their husbands were found to have elevated levels of paranoia, interpersonal sensitivity, and hostility, as well as loneliness, impaired marital and family relations, and lack of social support." ("From Front Line to Home Front: A Study of Secondary Traumatization - 552b8a780cf2e089a3 aa40ec.pdf,")

Whereas the prior study did not provide prevalence statistics of Secondary PTSD among wives of combat Veterans, the following study noted that:

".. . half of the wives of war veterans with PTSD had 6 or more symptoms of secondary traumatic stress. Only 3 did not have any of the symptoms. Previous studies that investigated the causes of secondary traumatization in wives of Israeli veterans with PTSD, Dutch veterans, and Vietnam war veterans found that the mental and physical health condition of the person that suffered a direct trauma influenced the mental and physical health of the person providing support, and that veterans' wives manifested a wide range of mental and physical symptoms corresponding to the symptoms of PTSD.

"Koić et al. found that one third of wives (30%) of veterans diagnosed with PTSD met the criteria for secondary traumatic stress. Our study results not only confirmed the findings reported by these authors, but showed that even a larger proportion (39%) of veterans' wives suffered from secondary traumatic stress." (Frančišković et al., 2007)

Among professionals such as policemen, EMS, nurses, etc., a term called Compassion Fatigue emerged in the 1950's to initially describe these phenomena in nurses related to a loss of nurturing ability, particularly within emergency room settings. This condition involves a gradual lessening of compassion for others over a period of time.

Symptoms begin to mirror those evidenced in trauma-involved others including a persistent negative attitude that insures increasing levels of tension and conflict. Ultimately, the effect can extend into the workplace if the caretaker has become the primary source of financial support and is also employed outside of the home. Within the home, self-doubt, feelings of inadequacy as well as focusing difficulty begin to emerge. In my mind, the 'poison' has spread and Compassion Fatigue/PTSD has laid claim to another soul.

As you note in my earlier comments, I view these conditions as being the same. As I see it, the poison emanates from the primary carrier and then extends outward to those who are close to the afflicted person.

Some people perceive of this as a virus. I have referred to the p---ed off cobra's poison as an image that was seared into my mind when reported to me by an older combat Veteran.

Our next topic is not an easy one to discuss. A consequence of a chronic state of fight, flight or freeze is a diminished sexual drive that produces avoidance of sexual intimacy for too many. The energy associated with the sexual drive doesn't simply disappear. We can thank Sigmund Freud for his insights in this regard.

Unfortunately, this 'libidinal' energy (thank Sigmund again) has the capacity to turn into violent expression either against the self or, it becomes redirected towards others. The term, Intimate Partner Violence (IPV), encompasses the transformation of sexual energy into that of violent expression against the mate/companion and other close associates or former colleagues.

****

If you don't hear from me in the next 24 hours, call the police," she whispered, then hung up. My phone read 2:12 am; it was the third call in as many minutes. I tried calling back—no answer. I went back to sleep, angry at Kristi for calling in the middle of the night and scaring me with a single sentence.

The next morning I fired off an email: 'I cannot, for the love of God, imagine what you were thinking when you called last night. Please tell me.' Kristi and I had become battle buddies at home while our husbands were serving in Iraq in 2004-05.

We had cried each time a military family member called with word of a soldier's death or suicide; we grieved at funerals and gravesites, marches and memorials. We wept with and for each another when she or I learned that our husband had been mobilized for another deployment, and again when they finally came home.

Her husband had served three combat tours since 2002. The last one was the shortest yet, a mere 10 months, and Kristi wrote in an email that 'he actually came back pretty normal this time!' That was nearly four months ago. When my phone rang in the afternoon early last fall, I saw that it was her, and picked up.

Mark tried to strangle me last night, she blurted out. I called you from the bathroom. I locked myself in with the pets. I didn't want him to hurt my puppy. I'm sorry I called. I was just so scared, and I didn't have anyone else to call. I couldn't call the cops. (Bannerman, 2010)

****

The US Department of Veterans Affairs, National Center for PTSD refers specifically to violence and aggression between intimate partners. They suggest that:

"IPV can include physical, sexual or psychological abuse or stalking. Acts of IPV range in how often they occur or how violent they are. It can happen to women or men who have intimate relationships with women, men or both. It can happen no matter your age, income, race, ethnicity, culture, religion, or disability.

". . . Among women Veterans receiving health care in VA, between 3 to 7 of every 10 (or 30% to 70%) report having experienced IPV at some point in their lives. In active duty women, more than 3 in every 10 (or 36%) report having experienced one or more types of IPV during their service." ("Intimate Partner Violence - PTSD,")

We should be absolutely stunned at figures such as these. We send our daughters off to serve and not only are they in harm's way by the enemy but also by those who serve with them and are predatory to them.

Ultimately, when things go horribly wrong, many spouses of our active duty members or our Veterans decide that enough is enough. When the non-afflicted spouse is forced to face the reality of her/his being gradually poisoned by the cobra's venomous influence they may decide to end the relationship.

To save families, we must transform this position. We must say to our leaders inside and outside of our government that: enough is enough: send our sons and daughters home intact. It can and must be done. The following author informs us that:

"The divorce rate among military couples has increased 42 percent throughout the wars in Afghanistan and Iraq . . . adding to the woes of U.S. military veterans returning from the Middle East who already have to tackle war-related problems like post-traumatic stress disorder and high unemployment rates.

"Couples' plans to pursue divorce gain plausibility with each subsequent month a service member is deployed, according to new research by Family Life. . . The first 90 days after deployment are the most critical for military marriages, the organization says.

"'That window is the proven time frame during which people develop habits and set the tone for the future of their marriage. It's critical for military couples to establish healthy habits quickly as they struggle to reconnect and restructure their families,'

Family Life Founder and President Dennis Rainey said in a statement.

"Some of the most common issues touching fresh veterans are a rushed transition to civilian life, renegotiating roles with the partner, realizing both spouses have changed during deployment, and possibly the influence of post-traumatic stress disorder, the organization claims." ("Divorce Rate Among Afghanistan, Iraq War Vets Increases by 42 Percent (VIDEO),")

Might it be possible that the experience of falling in love, engaging in combat activity and being married are incompatible? Or alternatively, might the fly in the ointment be the presence of PTSD? When this factor enters the picture, it is likely that marital bliss become transformed into one of Alfred Hitchcock's horror movies. The following authors found that:

"Post-9/11 veterans who were married while they were in the service also had a more difficult time readjusting to life after the military. Overall, being married while serving reduces the chances of an easy re-entry from 63% to 48%.

At first glance, this finding seems counter-intuitive. Shouldn't a spouse be a source of comfort and support for a discharged veteran? Other studies of the general population have shown that marriage is associated with a number of benefits, including better health and higher overall satisfaction with life. The following author seeks to answer the question with the following comment:

"In fact, the answer to another survey question points to a likely explanation. Post-9/11 veterans who were married while in the service were asked what impact deployments had on their relationship with their spouse. Nearly half (48%) say the impact was negative, and this group is significantly more likely than other veterans to have had family problems after they were discharged (77% vs. 34%) and to say they had a difficult re-entry.

". . . Taken together, these findings underscore the strain that deployments put on a marriage before a married veteran is discharged and after the veteran leaves the service to rejoin his or her family." (Crenshaw,)

****

I deployed with a guy whose break-up with his wife was like a slow-motion car wreck, compounded by his total naivety and denial. First, she made "friends" with this Marine on base, then she gave away her husband's dog, then she withdrew $5,000 from their bank account.

"All the while he refused to see what was happening. Only after his wife's new Marine friend was arrested (for a sexual assault) did she call her husband and tell him. While he was on the phone with her in the middle of the shop with everyone there. All we heard was his end and it was devastating. "Did you sleep with him?" he asked. "Do you love him?" He got off the phone and tries to leave the building, but collapses in the hallway just outside the doorway and screamed, 'SHE F----- HIM!!!'

"We literally had to drag him back in the office before the majors and colonels who worked in our building came out to investigate, which they inevitably did. It was maybe the most ridiculous and dramatic thing I've ever seen, played out over three or four months in the deserts of Afghanistan. Really easy to predict, really hard to watch." (Katzenberg, 2015)

****

There is little question that emotional problems complicate marital or couples' reintegration of military service members after a wartime deployment. What is glaringly missing from this awareness is the vital discussion related to the causation factor that transforms a loving, kind, gentle person into a hardened, hyperalert, hyper-aroused individual who is in a chronic state of protect/defend.

Johnny goes marching off to war 'leaving his innocence behind him.' If we had a way to 'detox' him before he came home on his rotation or transition into civilian life, might we save marriages? I have no doubt that this would be the case. It wouldn't be that hard to do. Perhaps a one or two hour meeting with a therapist utilizing neurotherapeutic interventions could make all the difference in the world.

After Johnny's 'kill switch' is turned off, he leaves his aggressive persona behind him until his next combat tour, when his survival needs kick in the switch again. Is this far-fetched? I don't think it is.

Therapists are experiencing difficulties in dealing with couple's issues in returning Veterans. Is it any wonder? Someone different comes home and the civilian spouse is simply supposed to 'suck it up?' It doesn't seem that this strategy is working? As Dr. Phil is inclined to say, "How well is that working for you?"

Neither is the strategy that the issue is a communication problem between the couple. Problematic marriages or relationships always have a third element that weakens the bond. A classic example is that of the husband, wife and alcohol. Have you ever wondered why many beer bottles are vaguely shaped like a female form – a slim one at that?

Triangles in relationships are inherently unstable. When Johnny brings home PTSD as a house guest, a terrible destructive process begins ultimately destroying the fragile alliance that began on the wedding day. Now mind you, if the Veteran does not come home with PTSD, the adjustment process may still be difficult.

****

I spent almost an entire summer at sea on my ship completing pre-deployment work-up training. After the third and final certification exercise, I called my boyfriend, Tim, a Marine pilot, delighted to be on dry land and hoping to meet up before I finally left for block leave and deployment.

After reaching voicemail, Tim called me back while I was enjoying a margarita with one of my friends at a local Mexican restaurant. When I told him that yes, I was with company, he said, "Oh good, you're with someone who can take care of you after I tell you this news. I met a girl a week ago and I think she's the one. And besides, you're going to be gone a lot. I know this is probably pretty callous, but I hope you'll be happy for me.

. . .Well, you know I was never really going to 'come around' to you. I am so annoyed that you thought I would. By the nature of calling this a breakup, we've failed at what this should have been. I'll always value you as a friend. As it turned out, Tim did me a favor: I met my partner almost exactly six months later. (Katzenberg, 2015)

****

After the hugs and kisses, he comes in the door and begins the process of assuming his natural place in the hierarchy as the 'leader of the pack.' However, without the presence of PTSD, communication between two people still becomes possible. It may be difficult and some may fail, but at least there's a chance for compromise and adjustment. The following author reports that:

"Couples in which one spouse has recently returned from military deployment in Iraq or Afghanistan and are experiencing marital problems can present a significant treatment challenge. There is little empirical evidence regarding effective treatments for this population, and these couples tend to exhibit a wide range of difficulties, including the following: conflicts about reintegration, problems with posttraumatic stress disorder and/or depression, chronic injury, infidelity, and personal and social challenges associated with rejoining civilian life.

". . . ONE of the enduring effects of the controversial war in Vietnam has been an ever-increasing focus on the problems of military service members returning from a wartime deployment. The literature pertaining to this issue has expanded after every major military conflict or involvement since that time, including the first Gulf War, peace-keeping missions in Bosnia, and, most recently, the conflicts in Afghanistan (Operation Enduring Freedom [OEF]) and Iraq (Operation Iraqi Freedom [OIF]).

"In the wake of the OEF and OIF conflicts, we have another such painful opportunity to examine the impact of wartime deployment, problems in family reintegration after deployment, and our therapeutic methods of helping these families. Existing literature suggests that there is a negative impact of war on couples and family functioning.

"It is clear, however, that extended difficulty with family reintegration after wartime deployment is most acute when there are preexisting couple and family vulnerabilities as well as service member injury and psychiatric complications of combat." ("Family Reintegration Difficulties and Couples Therapy for Military Veterans and Their Spouses - Sayers 2011 Family reintegration difficulties and couples therapy for military veterans and their spouses.pdf,")

When Johnny is psychically cut off from himself, how is he is to have empathic sensitivity to those around him? He is numb to how his parents, spouse, children perceive of him because he is utterly locked in his world of protect and defend.

Unfortunately, entities and organizations that serve the Veteran come to expect the spouse to silently bear the burden of their disabled other because 'this is the honorable thing to do.' Through this mistaken message, shame is added to the burden. The authors of the following article advise that:

"Survivors with PTSD may feel distant from others and feel numb. They may have less interest in social or sexual activities. Because survivors feel irritable, on guard, jumpy, worried, or nervous, they may not be able to relax or be intimate. They may also feel an increased need to protect their loved ones. They may come across as increasingly tense or demanding.

"The trauma survivor may often have trauma memories or flashbacks. He or she might go to great lengths to avoid such memories. Survivors may avoid any activity that could trigger a memory. If the survivor has trouble sleeping or has nightmares, both the survivor and partner may not be able to get enough rest. This may make sleeping together harder.

"Survivors often struggle with intense anger and impulses. In order to suppress angry feelings and actions, they may avoid closeness. They may push away or find fault with loved ones and friends. Also, drinking and drug problems, which can be an attempt to cope with PTSD, can destroy intimacy and friendships. Verbal or physical violence can occur.

"In other cases, survivors may depend too much on their partners, family members, and friends. This could also include support persons such as health care providers or therapists.

"Dealing with these symptoms can take up a lot of the survivor's attention. He or she may not be able to focus on the partner. It may be hard to listen carefully and make decisions together with someone else.

Partners may come to feel that talking together and working as a team are not possible.

"Partners, friends, or family members may feel hurt, cut off, or down because the survivor has not been able to get over the trauma. Loved ones may become angry or distant toward the survivor. They may feel pressured, tense, and controlled. The survivor's symptoms can make a loved one feel like he or she is living in a war zone or in constant threat of danger.

"Living with someone who has PTSD can sometimes lead the partner to have some of the same feelings of having been through trauma.

"In sum, a person who goes through a trauma may have certain common reactions. These reactions affect the people around the survivor. Family, friends, and others then react to how the survivor is behaving. This in turn comes back to affect the person who went through the trauma." ("Relationships and PTSD - PTSD,")

As an insidious, toxic relationship develops, domestic violence surfaces too frequently. The following author addresses the presence of internalized anger in the form of self-destructive tendencies as well as violence directed towards the significant other.

"Combat veterans are responsible for almost 21 percent of domestic violence nationwide. . . This is comparable to the fact that veterans alone account for 20 percent of U.S. suicides. . . But we don't talk about veteran intimate partner violence at all, effectively ensuring that the catastrophic consequences remain largely unacknowledged and unaddressed.

"Even as the overall frequency of domestic abuse in the United States declined, levels of intimate partner violence within the post-9/11 military and veterans' communities began to explode. Calls from people affiliated with the military more than tripled from 2006 to 2011.

". . . Research has found that veterans diagnosed with PTSD were 'significantly more likely to perpetrate violence toward their partners,' with over 80 percent committing at least one act of violence in the previous year, and almost half at least one severe act, including strangulation, stabbing and shooting. This is more than 14 times higher than the general civilian population.

". . . Unlike typical civilian domestic violence, veteran intimate partner violence often . . . is an explosion of violence, rather than an escalation; there is typically no 'honeymoon' period after the event, as the veteran withdraws in shame; and the violence is more likely to be lethal or potentially lethal in severity.

". . . The confluence of unprecedented levels of traumatic brain injury, PTSD and other mental health disorders puts the post-9/11 generation of veterans at extremely high risk of perpetrating violence in the home." (Bannerman,)

****

A few months after Sgt. William Edwards and his wife, Sgt. Erin Edwards, returned to a Texas Army base from separate missions in Iraq, he assaulted her mercilessly. He struck her, choked her, dragged her over a fence and slammed her into the sidewalk.

As far as Erin Edwards was concerned, that would be the last time he beat her. Unlike many military wives, she knew how to work the system to protect herself. She was an insider, even more so than her husband, since she served as an aide to a brigadier general at Fort Hood.

With the general's help, she quickly arranged for a future transfer to a base in New York. She pressed charges against her husband and secured an order of protection. She sent her two children to stay with her mother. And she received assurance from her husband's commanders that he would be barred from leaving the base unless accompanied by an officer.

Yet on the morning of July 22, 2004, William Edwards easily slipped off base, skipping his anger-management class, and drove to his wife's house in the Texas town of Killeen.

He waited for her to step outside and then, after a struggle, shot her point-blank in the head before turning the gun on himself. ("When Strains on Military Families Turn Deadly - The New York Times,")

****

"Two-thirds of homeless Iraq and Afghanistan veterans in one major sample had post-traumatic stress disorder (PTSD) — a much higher rate than in earlier cohorts of homeless veterans. . . The high rates of PTSD make sense because all Iraq and Afghanistan veterans were deployed and many saw combat, while many of their counterparts of previous eras weren't deployed," says the study's lead author, psychologist Jack Tsai, PhD, of Yale University.

". . . In addition to combat-related PTSD, 7.7 percent of male homeless Iraq and Afghanistan veterans and nearly a quarter of female homeless veterans from these wars reported having PTSD that was related to previous traumas, which other studies show can include childhood abuse, assaults and rape. Furthermore, 15 percent of men and 34.1 percent of women in this sample who reported combat-related PTSD also reported PTSD that wasn't related to combat." ("More PTSD among homeless vets,")

****

When 'Iraqi Freedom' began, Private First Class Herold Noel was a soldier in the U.S. Army's 3rd Infantry Division, pounding a path into Baghdad. "I fought for this country," he said. "I shed blood for this country. I watched friends die." And like so many, Herold Noel came home a hero, but he wound up homeless.

When the war in Vietnam washed up the first wave of veterans in need of shelter -- the Department of Veteran Affairs had no homeless programs at all. While today, they offer services in every state. Still, as many as 275,000 veterans will likely sleep out in the cold tonight.

Herold was diagnosed with Post Traumatic Stress Disorder. Unemployed, married with three kids, he couldn't get a job. "The physical war is over. The mental war has just begun," he said.

. . . I put applications in. I did all that. They lost my application three f^&@# times!" Noel said. This time a city housing agency has given him the runaround yet again. 'What are you telling me man? I have three kids out there man! I fought for my country man. My country shouldn't be doing this to me."

Still, Herold Noel is one of the luckier ones. Just recently an anonymous donor heard Herold's story and is paying his rent for a year. Tonight, one Iraq War veteran is off the street. But somewhere soon, another could well take his place. (25, 2005, & Pm,)

****

Summary

I've developed this chapter from the perspective of a marital therapist trained in Family Systems Therapy. Since I view the family as the essential component for preparing our future citizens, my focus on this aspect of the 'system' attempted to address the negative change elements that trauma brings into the marriage/relationship.

While most of my discussion involves combat Veterans with PTSD, I could have just as easily substituted those who serve our communities in our emergency rooms, police and fire departments, etc. Trauma doesn't only occur on the battle field.

I discussed the wife, significant other, companion, etc., as the first 'clash point' with the outcome dependent upon the veracity? and coping ability of the initially non-traumatized mate. The parallel may be akin to those who tolerate spousal abuse, indeed they may come to experience Intimate Partner Violence. Another similar model may be found among those who are referred to as 'enablers' within the context of their alcoholic spouses.

These are folk that have been described as adaptive individuals who seek to adjust in order to better cope with the circumstances they find themselves in. Others who choose not to be so adaptive are likely to be among those who end up in the divorce court. These divergent pathways take their toll as the family executors either clash or one cedes power to the other.

When the marriage comes to an end, amid the carnage that's created, the PTSD involved Veteran more likely than not self-medicates and/or, engages in self-destructive ideation. When the Veteran hits bottom, for many, the street becomes their home. While enormous resources are going into ending homelessness among Veterans, the primary causative factor of PTSD remains untreatable through current methodologies.

Those that adapt are exposed to the toxicity of trauma's effects over extended periods. This may attain a level where many of the spouses lose their spontaneity and become protective/defensive of their own well-being. This occurs within the context of a weakening physical bond between those who previously shared moments of intimacy.

Gradually, the relationship shifts to that of a caretaker position. The hyperarousal of the Veteran permeates into all aspects of the couple's functioning. As one finds increasingly in the pattern of spousal abusers, others are cut progressively out of 'the circle of trust.' Isolation and withdrawal become central and foremost.

Numerous stories were provided in this chapter to illustrate the toxic effects that PTSD has on family structure. Rather than a stable unit, it becomes foundationally unstable. Rather than wisely guiding its offspring, the PTSD family becomes mired in its own toxicity. And what about the offspring? This subset will be the topic of our next chapter.

References

25, B. C.-M. C. M., 2005, & Pm, 4:29. From Hero To Homeless. http://www.cbsnews. com/news/from-hero-to-homeless/

Bannerman, S. (2010, September 25). Husbands Who Bring the War Home. http://www. thedailybeast.com/articles/2010/09/25/ptsd-and-domestic-abuse-husbands-who-bring-the-war-home.html

Bannerman, S.High risk of military domestic violence on the home front. http://www. sfgate.com/opinion/article/High-risk-of-military-domestic-violence-on-the-5377562.php

Crenshaw, E. The View from Someone Else's Boots,. http://blog.gettinghired.com/Home

/tabid/159/entryid/121/civilian-workplace-success-with-transitioning-veterans.aspx

Divorce Rate Among Afghanistan, Iraq War Vets Increases by 42 Percent (VIDEO). http://www.christianpost.com/news/divorce-rate-among-afghanistan-iraq-war-vets-hits-42-percent-66195/

Frančišković, T., Stevanović, A., Jelušić, I., Roganović, B., Klarić, M., & Grković, J. (2007). Secondary Traumatization of Wives of War Veterans with Posttraumatic Stress Disorder. *Croatian Medical Journal*, *48*(2), 177–184.

From Front Line to Home Front: A Study of Secondary Traumatization - 552b8a7 80cf2e089a3aa40ec.pdf. https://www.researchgate.net/profile/Zahava_Solomon/publication/21703493_From_Front_Line_to_Home_Front_A_Study_of_Secondary_Traumatization/links/552b8a780cf2e089a3aa40ec.pdf

Intimate Partner Violence - PTSD: National Center for PTSD. http://www.ptsd va.gov/public/types/violence/domestic-violence.asp

Katzenberg, L. (2015, February 13). Here Are 8 True Stories Of Awful Deployment Breakups. http://taskandpurpose.com/8-true-stories-terrible-deployment-breakups

More PTSD among homeless vets. http://www.apa.org/monitor/2013/03/ptsd-vets.aspx

Relationships and PTSD - PTSD: National Center for
    PTSD. http://www.ptsd.va.gov/
    public/family/ptsd-and-relationships.asp

Secondary PTSD. http://www.familyofavet
    .com/secondary_ptsd.html

Street, 1615 L., NW, Washington, S. 800, &
    Inquiries, D. 20036 202 419 4300 | M. 202
    419 4349 | F. 202 419 4372 | M. (2011,
    October 5). War and Sacrifice in the Post-
    9/11 Era. http://www.pewsocial trends.
    org/2011/10/05/war-and-sacrifice-in-the-post-
    911-era/

When Strains on Military Families Turn Deadly -
    The New York Times. http://www.nytimes
    .com/2008/02/15/us/15vets.html

Chapter Six

Rugrats

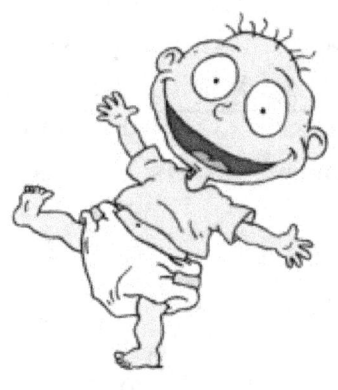

"Abuse manipulates and twists
a child's natural sense of trust and love.
Her innocent feelings are belittled or mocked
and she learns to ignore her feelings.
She can't afford to feel
the full range of feelings in her body
while she's being abused—pain, outrage, hate,
vengeance, confusion, arousal.
So she short-circuits them and goes numb.
For many children,
any expression of feelings,
even a single tear, is cause for more severe abuse.
Again, the only recourse is to shut down.
Feelings go underground."

Laura Davis, Allies in Healing

****

For much of the first year-and-a-half of young Christian Martinez' life, he only saw his mother, Technical Sgt. Caroline Martinez, on a laptop screen as they Skyped from half a world away. When she returned in 2010 for a 15-day leave toward the end of her one-year deployment . . . her son was confused.

The first time he looked at me, I don't think he recognized me entirely," Martinez said. "My husband kept saying, "This is mom. Mom." And he went to the laptop, and tapped on the laptop, and said, "Mom." I said, "No, I'm Mom."

Since then, said Martinez, . . . she and Christian have been "joined at the hip." That was by far the hardest of her five deployments. These days, when Martinez deploys, it's only for about four months at a time, giving her plenty of time to take now-7-year-old Christian to soccer games and be involved in his other extracurricular activities.

Martinez isn't alone. According to deployment statistics provided by the Air Force, tens of thousands of airmen are still deploying these days — but the pace is declining from a few years ago, when the Afghanistan surge was at its peak.

. . .While fewer airmen are deploying, the average number of days that those who do deploy spend overseas has increased. In 2013, enlisted airmen deployed for 110 days on average. . . But in 2015, the average enlisted airman deployed for 132 days . . . a little more than six months. (Times,)

****

Too many of the children of our combat servicemen and Veterans have been exposed to an invisible and emotional form of viral infestation called PTSD. Some perceive that it is transmitted through modeling within the family context. Others see it as a change in the genetic structure of the afflicted individual that can be transmitted through multi-generations. Whatever the causation, it's time for us to address it. It's time for us to stop it!

An assistant professor at the Virginia Tech Carilion Research Institute, studied the effect that observing fear in others might have on physically changing the structure of the brain. Alexei Morozov, the lead author of the study tells us that:

"... the part of the brain responsible for empathizing and understanding the mental state of others . . . physically changes after witnessing fear in another. . . And this redistribution is achieved by stress . . . through social cues, such as body language, sound, and smell." ("Witnessing fear can physically change the brain, say Virginia Tech Carilion Research Institute scientists,")

Scientists at the U.S .Department of Veterans Affairs, National Center for PTSD, discuss the development of the brain in the young while under stress. This is a time of rapid development that is partially shaped by experience. The researchers tell us that "Prolonged stress can lead to increased arousal, elevated stress hormones, and biochemical alterations of emotion regulation circuits.

"In essence, early stress and trauma can alter the brain and have long-term effects across many domains, including physical, mental, and emotional development. Moreover, the impact of early maltreatment often extends into later childhood, adolescence, and even adulthood." ("Trauma, PTSD, and Attachment in Infants and Young Children - PTSD,")

The end result transforms the child from a perspective of growing and being curious to one of 'protect and defend.' Earlier, I discussed Secondary

166

Trauma. Some of the vignettes provided in this chapter illustrate both the process and destructive outcome for those children who are vulnerable to the damaging exposure. A number of the stories I've included are at the extreme end of the spectrum to help you understand what occurs when things go terribly wrong.

****

Brannan and Katie's teacher have conferenced about Katie's behavior many times. Brannan's not surprised she's picked up overreacting and yelling—you don't have to be at the Vines residence for too long to hear Caleb hollering from his room, where he sometimes hides for 18, 20 hours at a time, and certainly not if you're there during his nightmares, which Katie is.

"She mirrors…she just mirrors her dad's behavior," Brannan says. She can't get Katie to stop picking at the sores on her legs, sores she digs into her own skin with anxious little fingers. She is not, according to Brannan, "a normal, carefree six-year-old." ("Is PTSD Contagious? | Mother Jones,")

****

Clearly, the lifestyle of the military family differs from their civilian counterparts. A *Los Angeles Times*, January 30, 2017 article focused on differences between our military and civilian populations. The reporters suggest that multigenerational families form "the heart of the all-volunteer Army."

They comment that a shrinking percentage forms the conscription pool and that four out of five who serve had a family member who was also in the military. Furthermore, they tend to be isolated from the surrounding civilian population due to their residing in military installations. The reporters note that:

"The segregation is so pronounced that it can be traced on a map: Some 49% of the 1.3 million active-duty service members in the U.S. are concentrated in just five states — California, Virginia, Texas, North Carolina and Georgia. The U.S. military today is gradually becoming a separate warrior class, many analysts say, that is becoming increasingly distinct from the public it is charged with protecting.

"Most of the country has experienced little, if any, personal impact from the longest era of war in U.S. history. But those in uniform have seen their lives upended by repeated deployments to war zones, felt the pain of seeing family members and comrades killed and maimed, and endured psychological trauma that many will carry forever, often invisible to their civilian neighbors." ("U.S. military and civilians are increasingly divided - LA Times,")

To briefly summarize at this point, we have a selective pool of future members of our military who are drawn from around 80% of those of their elders, many who have previously served. By extension, let's assume that around 50% of those in that selection pool have PTSD. This is a fair approximation of the post-9/11 statistics. Are we thus recycling this disturbance through a small part of our population?

Because of the limited pool that our all-volunteer armed forces are being drawn from and the shrinking size of the force, increased levels of rotation into combat theaters have become the routine rather than the exception. With the PTSD recycling effect as discussed above, frequent deployment appears to be associated with increasing levels of maltreatment and neglect among younger military related children as noted in the following discussion:

"Another term in use for the time spent at home is 'Dwell Time.' The first study to compare the emergence of mental health issues within the context of the military rotation cycle in regards to time spent at home came up with some interesting findings. The researchers found that the rates of PTSD were consistent with other studies however, PTSD rates were elevated when two or more employments occurred. Longer 'dwell times' seemingly lowered the rates in a reciprocal manner." ("America's Medicated Army, 2.0 | TIME.com,")

****

Her father's despair seeped into every waking moment, poisoning the family. By age 5, Christal Presley routinely barricaded her dresser against her bedroom door. He could go from fetal position to fury. "I'm going to the river, and I won't be back!" he would yell, grabbing a gun.

"For the first two years of that, I was especially traumatized, and I was afraid he was not coming back," Presley, now 35, said of her father, who threatened to kill himself twice a week. "As a young teenager, I used to pray that he would just do it." When you grow up with that, you're faced with that fight-or-flight feeling every single day.

It would be years before the source of her terror had a name: PTSD. And it was hers — for having grown up subjected to her Vietnam vet father's post-traumatic stress disorder.

Presley thought, "That's crazy, how can I have symptoms of a war I never fought in?"

. . . Presley recalls being in kindergarten when her father snapped. He was on the road to work when he came upon his co-worker and best friend in the world, dead in his truck.

"He stayed locked in his room after that. He was mostly lying on his bed, in a fetal position," recalled Presley, "and when he came out of his room, he was very easily agitated; if a truck backfired down the road, or a plate or glass broke, he would fall down on the floor in war mode. . . I just was never sure what he'd do next." ("PTSD Haunts Children of Vets," 2014)

****

I'd like to further explore the deployment cycle that involves the entire family including their routines, emotional highs and lows, and stability or loss of it. For those who have made military service a career, this pattern of life has become routine. For those left behind, another type of routine takes place where the family members, who remain at home, shift to a different type of single-parent system.

For many of these families, the most difficult time in the cycle is when the absent parent comes home. They have learned to handle the long period of separation and look forward to the missing parent's return. When he/she comes back, the family system must shift again and those who are at home take on new roles. The rhythm and beat of the family once again alters.

Deployment typically is understood to consist of five stages including the following: 1) Pre-deployment, 2) Deployment, 3) Sustainment, 4) Redeployment, 5) Reintegration. Different definitions of this process are being considered but basically, the above description will suffice at this time. I will briefly describe each of these stages in regards to the typical impact it may have on the child. I'd like to credit the webpage, Military Kids Connect, for a number of the ideas I've included in this chapter.

The first stage (Pre-deployment) begins with the gradual warning and emerging awareness which finally becoming a firm order to deploy. With the actual departure, this stage is ended. This period can be a few weeks to upwards of one year.

Involvement in training typically occupies the military member in activities such as field training and an increase in activity away from the home. The primary focus is to keep the skills of war sharpened for use when the next assignment is called for. During this period, the family system shifts in an effort to accommodate the returned military member.

This is often confusing for young children (0-5) who constitute about 40% of the family membership. As the departure time draws near, the soldier enhances his 'bond' and time with other members of his unit to establish the cohesion necessary for combat activity. Unfortunately, his 'bond' to his family as well as time spent with them weakens accordingly.

To-do lists are accomplished one by one. Concerns about the upcoming separation are hopefully addressed. The stay at home parent begins the shift to her/his home single parent status. Unfinished personal business is often missed with hurts and misunder-standings accruing.

As the departure date approaches, arguments may increase both in frequency and intensity reflecting the underlying emotional upheaval leading up to the actual departure. Stoking anger may be a survival mechanism for the soldier to return to a world of danger once again.

For the spouse, it becomes a hard way to say goodbye. For the children, it becomes a fearful time filled with uncertainty and conflicts demonstrated in the parents. For younger children, regressive behavior may be evidenced both in mood and behavior.

****

We've gotta be ready for anything," my father said to me when I was 12 as he packed the trunk . . . with camping supplies—a tent, emergency ponchos, hunting knives, blankets, boots, socks, gloves, a waterproof sleeping bag, several gallons of water, and a box full of freeze-dried army rations.

He'd accounted for everything we'd need for a week long camping trip in a remote jungle location completely cut off from society. Except we weren't going camping . . . We were going to dinner at Chili's in suburban Philadelphia."

When we got to the restaurant, we had to wait until the 'good booth' in the corner was available before we sat down—the booth where my father could sit, his back to the wall with a clear sightline of all exits and entrances.

"That way no one can jump out at you," he'd say with a smile, like he was joking. . . I smiled back, just hoping we could get through the meal without him exploding with rage over undercooked food or a slow waiter or me.

He wanted me sitting 'at attention'—back straight, not slouched, feet flat on the floor, napkin across lap. No fidgeting. No elbows.

. . . I'm 40 now and I've been battling my father's Vietnam ghosts my whole life. . . My son is nine months old now and I hope it's not too late for me to avoid passing this trauma on to him. Forty years at war is more than enough. I am ready for peace. ("I Inherited My Dad's PTSD,")

****

The second phase of the cycle (deployment) involves the actual movement of the troops from their home settings to the operating theatre. This might be stateside or abroad. Upon arrival, the troops engage in their specified mission maintaining their fighting and support related skills.

During the deployment period, adjustment to the change in the system takes place bringing with it both positives and negatives. The ability to communicate is generally a positive thing in that it established a lifeline between the family and the soldier.

Alternatively, this same connection can further intensify unresolved feeling and unfinished business.

Hearing about some of the children acting out, others withdrawing, etc., doesn't exactly produce an 'Ozzie and Harriet' moment. In a similar vein, the call home has typically been limited to fifteen minutes. Changes have been made thanks to cell-phones that have altered this limitation.

Being in a place of danger adds to the stress level. The service member tries to filter out disturbing experiences he has been involved in however, the feeling channel of our communication system conveys the message independent of the verbal denial.

During the deployment period, babies and toddlers are highly reactive to their surroundings. The bonding with the primary caretaker has likely becomes more intense after one of the parents leaves.

Confusion is more likely to be expressed in the toddler. Clinging behavior may be evidenced. At this stage, degrees of anger may be expressed including temper tantrums. They will also copy the behaviors and emotions of the primary parent.

Pre-schoolers may self-blame and/or worry about the remaining parent in regards to fear of losing them too. They like routine and tend to stay close to the primary caretaker. Behavioral difficulties may be expressed in loss of interest in food, bedwetting or potty accidents. They may act out frightening experiences as part of their play. Outbursts, tantrums and aggressiveness may also be present.

School age children sense a vacuum within the family structure following the departure of the service member. Children in this age group are also inclined to worry and fret about the parent who may be in harm's way. To add to their concern, they may fear that the primary parent will abandon them as well.

Some of the older kids including the teenagers may step in assuming the role of parental children. They attempt to assist the remaining parent taking the role of mom or dad. If this is encouraged and rewarded, and then criticized when the absent parent returns, confusion and resistance takes place.

From the negative perspective, many children in this age group may develop physical symptoms such as headaches and stomach aches in reaction to changes in their routine. Changes in mood may also be evident. They will also seek to buffer stress from the remaining parent.

Alternatively, they may act out in their effort to establish a balance between themselves and the adults within their lives. They may also turn to their peers for guidance as an alternative to the remaining, overwhelmed parent.

Stage 3 (Sustainment) is the period in which the service member continues to engage in the assigned duty of the tour. I'd like to provide you with a little history of changes in deployment for many of our Post-9/11 service personnel that have dramatically changed the nature of military service.

"In March 2003, U.S. forces invaded Iraq in what became known as Operation Iraqi Freedom. American forces included both active duty and reserve forces. The original plan was for U.S. forces to be withdrawn quickly after hostilities had ended, much as they had in Desert Storm in the early 1990s. Indeed, by May 1, 2003, President Bush declared the end of major combat operations. But the planned decrease in the U.S. forces did not take place.

"An insurgent operation developed with increased sectarian violence as ethnic groups gained new freedom. To meet this new and prolonged threat, the U.S. military rotated units and even individual service members, both active and reserve, serving in Iraq. Today some soldiers and Marines are on their third, fourth, and even fifth rotation.

"Over time, the frequency of deployments and the time between deployments, or dwell time as it has become known, has become a point of deep concern both in and outside the military. What impact will the frequent deployments and short dwell times have on the morale and health of both active and reserve soldiers and their families? ("untitled - ADA478163.pdf,")

The remainder of this chapter will focus on an attempt to answer that question. The following material is taken from a webpage entitled "Army Sustainment – Professional Bulletin of United States Army Sustainment – Challenges to Maintaining Readiness in a Deployed Environment," by Major Terry D. Brannan, who informs us that:

". . . battlefield losses can impact unit effectiveness and lower morale. . . The 10th Sustainment Brigade's deployed permanent loss statistics were surprising. From December 2008 through the end of August 2009, pregnancy, family issues, and misconduct or legal problems constituted 60 percent of the brigade's personnel losses.

"Eighty-seven percent of those who left for those reasons were in the rank of staff sergeant or below. The family issues tracked for this statistic included failed family care plans, financial issues that arose because of inadequate preparation, lack of family preparedness, and repeated misconduct of family members.

"In contrast, the 10th Sustainment Brigade's casualty losses were just 1 percent of the total personnel losses, even though the brigade spent its entire 12-month deployment supporting the Multi-National Division-Baghdad area of operations.

"It may be impossible to entirely avoid losses caused by pregnancy, family issues, and misconduct or legal problems. However, commanders' and S–1s' consistent and thorough application of existing doctrine and regulations for pre-deployment readiness can substantially reduce the occurrence of these types of losses." ("Army Sustainment: Challenges to Maintaining Readiness,")

I'd like to offer an interpretation of the above material provided by Major Brannan. It is clear that casualty losses sustained during the specified employment constituted 1% of total personnel losses. Another 60% of loss is due to interpersonal, family related matters including "repeated misconduct of family matters."

It appears to me that things aren't going too well on the home front based on these figures. Supposedly, during this period, the family at home reaches out to available sources of support including extended family, friends, church or other support networks. Theoretically, as challenges arise, the spouse is supposed to learn to cope with crises and make important decisions on her own. Apparently, this isn't working. Why?

I'll try to answer that question by providing a bit of a conspiracy theory. A small group in our population (0.5%) are recycling a form of 'mental virus' to another small group (0.6%) who they leave behind while they engage in military and support operations. The home-based group pick up the virus and spread it among themselves each time the military member returns from multiple tours back to the home. The result of the virus leads to increasing levels of isolation and cutoff from others in their extended family and former support network.

As the virus takes hold, personalities change, conflict between family members ensues, acting-out behavior occurs. None of the currently available therapeutic interventions are able to block the spread of this disturbance. As it spreads, the efficiency and effectiveness of our armed forces diminishes accordingly. Well, that's only a hypothetical, or is it?

****

Tara and Russ Edwards have three children, Drew (23), Jordan (19) and Brennyn (8). They live in Anchorage, Alaska, where Russ has been stationed for the past 21 years. Now a search-and-rescue pilot, Russ has served in Turkey, in Kuwait and twice in Afghanistan since 9/11.

". . . When he first went over, he was allowed one phone call for 15 minutes every week, and he'd have to call command post first. Now Russ is able to email and make phone calls more regularly through a computer on base," she said.

. . . For the Edwardses, this has translated into emotional issues for Brennyn and problems with authority at one point for Drew. Tara said Brennyn would cry and say, "I miss my dad," while Drew would take issue with simple routines, such as being picked up from school.

"One time after Russ was deployed, I went to pick Drew (he was in 9th grade) up from school and I remember him saying, 'I didn't tell you to pick me up ... I want to spend time with my friends—I'm not getting in the car,'" Tara said.

(Tara) "You get into a routine, figure it all out, and then when he gets home, feelings get hurt or he may not think I was doing certain things right." Throughout the reintegration process, the Edwards family has relied on their church community for support.

"I remember asking people specifically to pray for that re-entry time," Tara said. "If the kids were doing things that were acceptable for a few months, and he's been with adults and on his own schedule, sometimes the kids would be too noisy, or when toys weren't put away, he may get mad. ("Military children bearing the stresses of war, reintegration,")

****

I will address the effects of a prolonged Sustainment period. With the onset of depression or other mental conditions in the primary at-home caretaker, a direct effect on the at-risk status of the infant occurs. Among other reactions in a previously thriving child are apathy, loss of appetite and consequent weight loss.

Toddlers are highly sensitive to the primary caretaker. If the parent is not coping well, the youngster might respond with an array of behavioral responses including: sleep disturbance, excessive demands for nurturing, temper tantrums and regressive behaviors. Preschoolers may evidence similar regressive behaviors such as clinginess, requests to sleep with the primary parent, irritability, body symptoms such as 'tummy aches.'

School age children may evidence depressive symptoms including withdrawal from peer contacts, slippage in school grades, aggressive outbursts that include acting out of their inner feelings. In a similar fashion, teenagers may engage in varied and unpredictable attention getting behavior.

Of course, their difficulties tend to be a magnification of symptoms evidenced in their younger peers. Their experimentation may also involve promiscuity, drug and alcohol use.

Stage 4 (Post-Deployment) is the return to home period with your soldier preparing to re-engage back into the world he had left behind. This would be an ideal time to utilize interventions that would defuse internal turmoil created by traumatic experiences within the tour.

Unfortunately, no such intervention is in current use. Counseling may be provided for some however, it does not 'reset the fear switch' prior to the soldier's actual physical contact with his family. The critical moment is lost to block the family infestation that will certainly occur when Johnny brings PTSD home with him.

Post-Deployment is defined as a phase where the service member reintegrates into 'normal life.' How can this be possible when he comes home in a 'protect and defend' state of mind? How can his varied briefings, training, medical evaluations, etc., prepare him for 'normal work' at the installation when he is no longer normal?

Finally, we reach stage 5, (Reintegration) that includes the service member becoming a part of the family and community once again. Struggles may ensue as each member finds their position again in the reformed family unit.

The following vignette is about Lt. Col. Michael Jackson, who retired from the US Air Force after 22 years of service including three deployments and his wife, who supported his family while he served.

****

I have a 2-year-old and a 2-week-old, and my husband won't be home . . . I was afraid the whole time. It lasted about four months. . . The next one came in July 2008, again to Afghanistan.

. . . His first day in the country followed an attack that killed several American service members. "Everything got a lot more real," he said. "My sense of vulnerability went up."

The situation didn't bode well for Anne Jackson. . . The water heater flooded . . . The garbage disposal broke. . . "There was a point . . . when I started to cry and couldn't stop," she said.

. . . 'You get back here, and it's just chaos everywhere,' said Michael Jackson, referring to the stark contrast between home life and a military deployment, where everything is structured . . .'He didn't adjust well . . . He withdrew,' Anne Jackson said. 'He would sit and watch TV.'

The third deployment came 18 months later . . . this time to Iraq with a Special Forces unit. . . . His wife broke her wrist while riding a bicycle. The toilet overflowed on New Year's Eve. The family dog died.

When Michael returned . . . we were all happy; but within weeks, we were all struggling . . . This eventually led me to really watch Michael's behavior to try and see what was going on — what the disconnect was. ("Studying military families," 2016)

****

Seemingly, the Reintegration period (Dwell Time) is the most difficult of all. Recall that Lt. Col. Jackson served three tours over a career period of 22 years. This is no longer the case in the Post-9/11 period. Deployments occur more frequently. The following authors inform us that:

"According to the Department of Defense, as of June 30, 2011, 203,400 military personnel . . .were currently on deployment in Iraq or Afghanistan. As nearly one half of all military personnel are parents, and with almost two million children having a military parent, there are a growing number of families who are experiencing or have experienced the strain of wartime deployments.

". . . Reintegration can be a turbulent time for the family, as members must re-form into a functioning system. Some studies suggest that relationship stress and negative family function may reach a peak between 4 to 9 months after the service member's return. One of the greatest challenges for these families appears to be renegotiating family roles as the service member encounters the often-unexpected difficulty of fitting into a home routine that has likely changed a great deal since his or her departure.

"Typically, over the course of one or more deployments, the at-home parent and children (especially adolescents who are more capable of providing greater instrumental support within the home) assume new responsibilities such that when the service member returns, there may be expectations among family members that things will either return to how they were prior to deployment or that the structure that emerged during deployment will remain. Lack of appropriate expectations and communication around this restructuring is a frequent source of conflict and stress for reintegrating families." (Saltzman et al., 2011)

It seems that 'Dwell Time' (time at home) is a critical variable associated with the onset of mental health disorders such as PTSD. [need a segue here] When trauma interrupts the efficiency of the soldier in the operating field an apparent first solution is to medicate in order to sustain the troop level needed. The following vignette is an example of such a policy.

****

Seven months after Sergeant Christopher LeJeune started scouting Baghdad's dangerous roads — acting as bait to lure insurgents into the open so his Army unit could kill them — he found himself growing increasingly despondent.

. . . He recalls the order his unit got after a nighttime firefight to roll back out and collect the enemy dead. . . "You don't always know who the bad guys are," he says. "When you search someone's house, you have it built up in your mind that these guys are terrorists, but when you go in, there's little bitty tiny shoes and toys on the floor — things like that started affecting me a lot more than I thought they would.

So LeJeune visited a military doctor in Iraq, who, after a quick session, diagnosed depression. The doctor sent him back to war armed with the antidepressant Zoloft and the antianxiety drug clonazepam. "It's not easy for soldiers to admit the problems that they're having over there for a variety of reasons," LeJeune says. "If they do admit it, then the only solution given is pills." ("America's Medicated Army,")

****

I'd like to finish this chapter with a discussion of the impact that the returning serviceman has on the functioning of the family. Now imagine that it is Mark Trepanier (next vignette) coming home heavily medicated and clearly suffering from PTSD.

Upon his return home, his children are excited and happy. His school age children show a mixture of emotions including pride, confusion and later, some anger regarding his absence. They hesitate in reconnecting because of an unspoken fear of his leaving again.

After the initial welcome, filled with happiness, his teenagers have difficulty in quickly adapting to his return. One of them is quite indifferent and somewhat withdrawn. Everyone is sensitive to how he will take his place in the family again.

He experiences flashback and nightmares about his past three deployments. In reaction, he pulls away from his family pulling himself into the all too familiar 'protect and defend' mode.

****

TOWSON, Md. – Mark Trepanier likes to spend time with the chickens he keeps in the back yard. "It's a barometer for my stress levels," he said. They're relaxing. Trepanier, a former military intelligence analyst, once made six figures working for a defense contractor, but he can no longer hold down a job.

. . . He needs a task list to remember to feed the dogs, to take care of the pets, to take the trash out," his wife Gayle said. Trepanier was diagnosed with post-traumatic stress disorder after serving in the first Gulf War, in Bosnia and in North Africa. When he came home in 2007, he was different as a husband and a father, his wife said.

. . . Fourteen-year-old Genna, the oldest of the Trepaniers' four children, remembers how her father used to be – and how he changed after his service. "We would always play games and stuff, and so he didn't do that as much," she said. "And he seemed more separated at times. And he'd get like really emotional."

Gayle Trepanier said their kids have been on an emotional roller coaster, each responding differently to dad's condition. "Kendrick, for example, will act out at school to the point where they thought he had ADHD, but it's emotional distress that was causing his outbursts and just unable to relax," she said. . . The entire Trepanier family is in counseling trying to learn how to deal with a very different dad. ("PTSD's 'secondary' victims,")

Summary

In a healthy parent/child system, the parents are the executors of the family business, discussing differences between them. While understanding that it is natural for their children to seek to divide them (triangulate), they do their best to address this. "Daddy, mommy said it was alright for me to sleep over at my friend's house so can I go now?" "I'll talk with your mom about this and will get back to you."

Introduce the effects of trauma into the mix and our family unit, the essential building block of our culture, transforms into the toxic, defensive/protective system that no longer is focused on the growth process. Others call it 'Secondary PTSD.' Through my eyes it's not secondary; I see no difference in the effects of the cobra's poison on the entire family system from its effects on the service member. I provide the following vignette as another extreme example of intergenerational transformation of the PTSD virus. We must find a way to block this insidious transmission.

****

"In 1979, I was nine years old. My father had been back from Vietnam for four years by this time and he took me to see a movie for the only time I've ever watched a movie in a theater with him. Apocalypse Now.

Now, obviously, a nine year old shouldn't be watching a movie so violent and over the top. But, I wasn't watching the movie. I watched my father's tears stream down his face during the entire movie. I watched him relive his time in Vietnam with every frame of the movie. He flinched at shots fired and gritted his teeth at the on-screen injuries.

By this time in his life, he was a functioning alcoholic and drug addict making a living as a weed and hash dealer. But for those three hours in that movie theater, he was a teenager watching his friends die, screaming as bullets ripped through flesh.

I wasn't his son, I was a buddy in his platoon trying to stay alive, just like him. He was coated in sweat and smelled like gas station hot dogs with onions. And I sat there, mesmerized.

Looking back, I believe I learned how not to cry that day. I learned how to be strong for myself. I turned ten that summer, an adult long before I should have been. . . Scott Brooks ("War-Related Intergenerational Post Traumatic Stress Disorder (PTSD),"

****

I've provided you with limited information about how the traumatized family effects its offspring often in an intergenerational manner. The touching story of the son of a Veteran who told us that: "my son is nine months old now and I hope it's not too late for me to avoid passing this trauma on to him" is heartfelt.

The astounding statistics provided by Major Terry D. Brannan related to permanent loss casualties brings the issue home. ". . . family issues, and misconduct or legal problems constituted 60 percent of the brigade's personnel losses. . . In contrast, the 10th Sustainment Brigade's casualty losses were just 1 percent of the total personnel losses, even though the brigade spent its entire 12-month deployment supporting the Multi-National Division-Baghdad area of operations."

We must and will find a way to terminate this horrible condition. I keep saying that we have the means. I repeat that there is now hope to end this horrible life of constant nightmares for those who suffer from PTSD. In the next chapter I will discuss one such step towards the resolution of this challenge.

References

America's Medicated Army, 2.0 | TIME.com. http://nation.time.com/2012/04/09/americas-medicated-army-2-0/

Army Sustainment: Challenges to Maintaining Readiness. http://www.alu.army .mil/alog /issues/JulAug11/challenges_readiness.html

I Inherited My Dad's PTSD. https://tonic.vice .com/en_us/article/i-inherited-my-dads-ptsd

Is PTSD Contagious? | Mother Jones. http://www. motherjones.com/politics/2013/01/ptsd-epidemic-military-vets-families

Military children bearing the stresses of war, reintegration. PTSD Haunt s Children of Vets. (2014, March 25). https://www.element behavioralhealth.com/trauma-ptsd/long-arm-of-ptsd-haunts-children-of-vets/

PTSD's "secondary" victims: the children of veterans. http://america.aljazeera. com/ watch/shows/america-tonight /articles /2014/7/9/ptsd-from-ptsd-someveteransakids showasecondarytraumaa0.html

Saltzman, W. R., Lester, P., Beardslee, W. R., Layne, C. M., Woodward, K., & Nash, W. P. (2011).

Mechanisms of Risk and Resilience in Military Families: Theoretical and Empirical Basis of a Family-Focused Resilience Enhancement Program. *Clinical Child and Family Psychology Review*, *14*(3), 213–230. https://doi.org/10.1007/s10567-011-0096-1

Studying military families: Joy of reunion challenged by reality of everyday life. (2016, February 18). http://www.navso.org/news/studying-military-families-joy-reunion-challenged-reality-everyday-life

Times, A. F. air-force-deployment-tempo-brings-new-kinds-strains. https://www.airforcetimes.com/articles/air-force-deployment-tempo-brings-new-kinds-of-strains

Trauma, PTSD, and Attachment in Infants and Young Children - PTSD: National Center for PTSD. http://www.ptsd.va.gov/ professional /treatment/children/trauma_ptsd_attachment.asp

untitled - ADA478163.pdf. http://www.acq.osd.mil/dsb/reports/ADA478163.pdf

U.S. military and civilians are increasingly divided - LA Times. http://www.latimes.com/nation/la-na-warrior-main-20150524-story.html

Witnessing fear can physically change the brain, say Virginia Tech Carilion Research Institute scientists. http://research.vtc.vt.edu/news

/2017/jan/04/witnessing-fear-can-physically-change-brain/

Chapter Seven

Veteran's Court

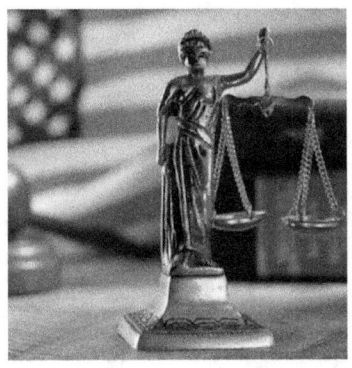

"I've learned, Agent Sanders,
most warriors feel the same way after they've
come back from the battles
where men in expensive suits
and leather chairs send them.
We keep asking and asking you to do the
impossible and even when you succeed
it seems the world doesn't change all that much.
Don't let that diminish your sacrifice,
and that of your family waiting at home.
Your country is proud of you."

C.J. Hatch

This chapter is focused on the recognition that our Veterans earned, through their service to this country, the right to a second chance. Implicit in this understanding is the recognition that a number of those Veterans who were affected by the horrors of war returned to civilian life as altered human beings.

A further extension of this understanding is the recognition that PTSD is a pervasive condition that negatively effects judgement, behavior and morality. To take this a step further, it is obvious that there is a strong association between PTSD and violent or antisocial behavior that may lead to legal ramifications and consequent incarceration among some of our veterans.

The framework for this chapter will be built on the rationale, indeed the absolute necessity leading to the creation of the Veteran's Court System. I will first make a case, pertaining to our Post-9/11 Veterans. Unfortunately, many of these individuals have had difficulties with reintegration into civilian society due to a high preponderance of trauma induced PTSD among this group. In this sense, they differ in the proportion of those with PTS from those who served before them.

A second presumption on my part, is that the causative factor for PTSD (trauma), is too often treated as a given that is an unchangeable constant.

What I mean by this is that we are inclined to accept the perspective that PTSD is a life-long condition that can be ultimately managed through ongoing medication and counseling but never fully remediated.

This way of thinking has pervaded the civilian population to the extent that when our veterans return to either re-integrate or touch base with their families on their varied rotations, others who come in contact with them perceive that they must be careful not to trigger the veterans' inner time bombs.

In contrast to this disheartening perspective, I will be building a case for adding a new type of treatment based on relatively recent advances in neuroscience. These innovations are capable of fully remediating the disruptive PTSD condition. When hope for a better life is restored, all things become possible.

The following research provides us with under-standing regarding the association between PTSD and violence in our Veteran and civilian population. The authors inform us that:

". . . the prevalence of violence among individuals with PTSD is 7.5% in the US population and 19.5% in post-9/11 Veterans. (This suggests that the association between PTSD and violence is especially strong in this Veteran cohort)." ("Research on PTSD, Aggression, and Violence – PTSD,")

There are many thoughts I have forthcoming from the violence numbers. One of them is that when we train people to kill and they return home unchanged with this demeanor, wouldn't we expect them to have difficulties with containing and restraining the emotions that accompany the behavior?

We expect the returning Veteran to leave the battlefield and automatically adjust back into the world of peace loving civilians. What a foolish assumption this is. I find it amazing that the incidence of violence isn't higher than the cited figures.

My training in Systems Family Therapy taught me to think in terms of three (triangle) which is considered to be the strongest geometric shape. When each of the sides is properly aligned, the shape is hard to distort because of the fixed angles and ability to distribute force evenly to each of the sides.

Of course, in family therapy, this is a metaphor for the family that can be utilized to diagram many aspects of their interaction such as the interactions between grandparents, parents and kids. It can also be utilized, outside of the family, to clarify specified components that support the continuance of an existing system.

I'll expound on this in my discussion of three critical points that in my mind, justified the emergence of an alternative judicial system referred to as a Veterans Treatment Court (VTC). The components are: 1) a societal trend for the incarceration of those with mental illness; 2) an increasing number of Veterans who have become homeless, and 3) an increase in the number of Veterans who have been sentenced in state and federal courts through the criminal court system. The author of the following article informs us that:

". . . prisons and jails have become America's 'new asylums.' Ten times more mentally ill people are now in jails and prisons than in state psychiatric hospitals: In 2012, approximately 356,268 inmates with severe mental illness were in prisons and jails, while about 35,000 severely ill patients were in state psychiatric hospitals.

". . . According to one report, the number of state psychiatric beds in the nation declined from a high of approximately 550,000 in 1960 to 40,000 today. So extremely sick people are locked up, often for trivial offenses, frequently without treatment, as their illnesses worsen. Upon release, they are more likely than other prisoners to recidivate and be incarcerated again." (Lithwick & Gillmor, 2016)

How is it that as a society we have turned our backs on the mentally ill and assigned them to poorly equipped law enforcement representatives to tend to them? Is this how our society is to be judged? To take it a step further, how can we possibly justify permitting seriously mentally ill persons to purchase firearms? I find myself asking who is insane in doing such a thing?

Perhaps it's easier to ignore than to address matters of such importance. While in state hospitals they were constrained to varying degrees and hopefully provided with some type of treatment. Now, too often, they are reprocessed through the revolving door of the court and prison systems. As to the second component of the triangle - homeless Veterans:

"The U.S. Department of Veterans Affairs (VA) states that the nation's homeless veterans are predominantly male, with roughly 9% being female. The majority are single; live in urban areas; and suffer from mental illness, alcohol and/or substance abuse, or co-occurring disorders. About 11% of the adult homeless population are veterans." ("National Coalition for Homeless Veterans,")

Additional information deriving from a 2014 report suggests that women constitute nearly 15% of our armed forces at present and will likely rise to around 19% among post-9/11 veterans. By 2020, the Department of Veterans Affairs expects female veterans to number more than 2 million which is about 10 percent of the veteran population.

". . . the fastest-growing segment of the homeless veteran population appears to be women, many of whom have children. Statistically, female veterans are between two and four times as likely as their civilian counterparts to become homeless, according to recent studies. And if they're young and black, those chances seem only to rise.

"Among these "new" homeless veterans, one risk factor stands out: a past history of sexual trauma — whether before, during or after military service, and sometimes all three.

"In a survey of the roughly 130,000 homeless veterans who used VA outpatient services in 2010, about 40 percent of the females, and 3 percent of the males, said they'd experienced military sexual trauma (MST)." ("The new face of veteran homelessness, by Lily Casura,")

The nature of PTS is to isolate and engage in protect and defend behaviors. The back against the wall phenomena is difficult for others to comprehend. It is unfortunate but understandable that family members find the returned Veteran's behavior peculiar or odd.

For some, significant others pull away and abandon their efforts to re-establish meaningful relationships with the altered person. They may reject the role of caretaker or, due to fear of potential harm, fully disengage from the afflicted individual.

Unable to sustain work due to varied factors including self-medicating, a number of our Veterans ultimately end up on the street, homeless and destitute. A number of them become the beggars that we encounter on the street corners of our communities. Others engage in criminal activity in order to sustain themselves.

The author of the following article provides us with the bricks and mortar for the final corner of our triangle, judicially treated Veterans. The author states that:

". . . After Vietnam, the number of inmates with prior military service rose steadily until reaching a peak in 1985, when more than one in five was a veteran. By 1988, more than half of all Vietnam veterans diagnosed with PTSD reported that they had been arrested; more than one third reported they had been arrested multiple times. Today veteran's advocates fear that, unless they receive proper support, a similar epidemic may befall soldiers returning from Iraq and Afghanistan." (Wolfe, 2013)

It is critical for us to understand the prevalence of those Veterans who are returning to a civilian world with PTSD. As discussed in prior chapters, having this condition, in and of itself, increases the likelihood of maladjustment and a general failure to smoothly transition back into the life of a citizen as opposed to that of a perpetual warrior.

A headline in the *Daily Beast* by Matthew Wolfe (07.28.13 4:45 AM ET) follows: "From PTSD to Prison: Why Veterans Become Criminals: Nearly one in 10 inmates have served in the military. The following story is one of many for those who served and are now imprisoned or have served time."

****

When Boyd drove, he watched the road for IEDs. The bombs could be disguised as almost anything; his team found them stashed in potholes, trash bags, and, once, in a dead sheep.

. . . Charlie Company received word that insurgent leaders were hiding in a house in a nearby town. . . Boyd steered a Humvee carrying nine members of his unit. When the soldiers arrived at the house, they found its front door open and no one home.

. . . Boyd hadn't moved 100 yards before he heard the explosion. . . Finally, the convoy started up again. . . when Boyd felt his vehicle shudder violently. . . Four of the Marines in the Humvee . . . were killed. Five others were injured. . . only Boyd escaped without injury.

A few months later, Boyd was back in Virginia, working a third shift at a Frito-Lay plant. He had trouble sleeping. . . he had nightmares about the raid. . . if he drank until he passed out, he didn't dream.

One Saturday morning in 2008, Boyd finished his shift and began to drink. . . The last thing Boyd says he remembers is sitting in the front seat of the car outside the party, drinking liquor.

When he woke up, he was in a police car, on his way to jail. The police officer told Boyd that he had shot his friend in the chest. The bullet made a clean exit, and the friend lived. Corporal Boyd was sentenced to five years in prison. ("From PTSD to Prison: Why

Veterans Become Criminals - The Daily Beast,")

****

I'll summarize the results of a 2010 study of a large group (1,543) of marines regarding antisocial tendencies among them. They had been deployed to combat zones in Iraq and Afghanistan during the 2002-2007 period. Five factors were explored that were thought to contribute to antisocial behavior. The study found that, "PTSD symptoms had a stronger association with antisocial behavior than any other variable." (Booth-Kewley, Larson, Highfill-McRoy, Garland, & Gaskin, 2010)

One might think that the above findings in a small group of combat marines isn't all that surprising. Another type of study called a meta-analysis took a look at 33 studies from 2007 to 2013 that involved the VA records of close to 5 million Operation Enduring Freedom and Operation Iraqi Freedom service members. The researchers came up with an estimate of 23% having PTSD among this group. (Fulton et al., 2015)

The above figure of 23% came from the review of notes in VA medical records but, how many of our Veterans actually use VA services? The National Center for Veterans Analysis and Statistics developed a 2014 Veteran profile that was published in May, 2016. They reported that: "As of 2014, there are 2.6 million Post-9/11 Veterans. As an end date to the Gulf War Era has not been established, the Post-9/11 cohort will continue to grow. VA projects a Post-9/11 Veteran population of just under 3.5 million by 2019."

The report further stated that only 37.3% of OEF/OIF Veterans enrolled in VA health care as compared to 46.5% per cent of other enrollees. Beyond enrollment, the actual use of VA services was found to be 19.9 percent among Post-9/11 Veterans as compared to 29.1 of other enrollees. ("Profile of Veterans: 2009 - Post_911_Veterans_Profile_2014.pdf,")

My understanding of the above material is that about 80% of Post-9/11 Veterans do not use VA health facilities at all. I find this to be rather stunning. Imagine, four out of five Veterans have nothing to do with a governmental health care agency that is supposed to care for them.

Why? Might it be part of their overall distrust of government in the first place? Might it be associated, at least partially, with the PTSD many carry home after engaging in modern warfare? To take this a step further, 70% of those who served before them also are inclined to avoid their involvement with the VA for their health care needs.

A CBS News blog published on October 5, 2011 headlined the story as follows: "Poll: 1 in 3 vets say Iraq, Afghan wars a waste." The reporter further states that:

"The poll results presented by the Pew Research Center portray post-Sept. 11 veterans as proud of their work, scarred by warfare and convinced that the American public has little understanding of the problems that wartime service has created for military members and their families.

"Nearly half of post-Sept. 11 veterans said deployments strained their relationship with their spouses, and a similar share reported problems with their children. . . Asked for a single word to describe their experiences, the war veterans offered a mixed picture: 'rewarding,' 'nightmare,' 'eye opening,' 'lousy.'" (5, 2011, & Am,)

It would be helpful if we knew what the true prevalence of PTSD was among our returning Vets. To clarify this important question further, I looked into two surveys that were conducted by the Pew Research Center comparing military veterans versus the general public. A total of 1,853 veterans were selected including 712 who served in the military after the 9/11/01 attacks. Results of the survey revealed that:

"44% of post-9/11 veterans say their readjustment to civilian life was difficult. By contrast, just 25% of veterans who served in earlier eras say the same. About half (48%) of all post-9/11 veterans say they have experienced strains in family relations since leaving the military, and 47% say they have had frequent outbursts of anger. One-third (32%) say there have been times where they felt they didn't care about anything.

"Nearly four-in-ten (37%) post-9/11 veterans say that, whether or not they were formally diagnosed, they believe they have suffered from post-traumatic stress (PTS). Among veterans who served prior to 9/11, just 16% say the same.

"These psychological and emotional problems are most prevalent among post-9/11 veterans who were in combat. About half of this group (49%) say they have suffered from PTS. And about half (52%) also say they had emotionally traumatic or distressing experiences while in the military. Of those who had these types of experiences, three-in-four say they are still reliving them in the form of flashbacks or nightmares." (Street, NW, Washington, & Inquiries, 2011)

You might be asking, what's the point here? The above information tells us that the range of Veterans reintegrating back into civilian life with PTSD ranges from 23% to upwards of 50%. With around 3 million Post-9/11 Veterans returning to civilian life, upwards of 1.5 million return with trauma related difficulties. With these figures, is it any wonder that:

"Of the homicides committed by OEF/OIF forces in the USA, one third of the victims were immediate family and one fourth were other members of the armed forces. Combat veterans are responsible for almost 21% of domestic violence calls nationwide and 20% of suicide calls.

"On the Domestic Violence Hotline, calls from military families tripled from 2006-2011, a time when abuse rates nationwide were declining. In one study, over 30% of a group of veterans diagnosed with PTSD self-reported committing at least one act of aggression in the previous year– mostly minor– but almost 11% self-reported at least one seriously violent act. Domestic abuse in the Army rose 177% from 2003-2010." ("Violence in Veterans, Fact or Fiction?," 2015)

I find these numbers to be quite startling. At its worst, half of those recent Veterans who return have serious PTS symptoms. One out of three homicides committed by those who served in the OEF/OIF era, were among immediate family members with 25% occurring with other service personnel.

David J. Morris wrote an article entitled: "War Is Hell, and the Hell Rubs Off: PTSD Contributes to Violence." He punctuates that: "Pretending it doesn't is no way to support the troops." David J. Morris an American writer and former Marine infantry officer who has come to challenge the 'Alternative Facts' pertaining to the relationship between PTSD and violence. He proposes that:

"The idea that PTSD is unrelated to violence back home is one of the central pillars of today's rigid 'support the troops' campaign. After every mass shooting event involving a veteran, Veterans Affairs psychiatrists and veteran's advocates deliver the same stern warning: Mentioning PTSD in conjunction with these shootings is not only inaccurate, it hurts veterans.

". . . The simple fact is that war poisons some men's souls, and we aren't doing our veterans any favors by pretending that war is only about honor and service and sacrifice and by insisting that PTSD is completely unrelated to the problem of postwar violence. It's not only morally irresponsible, it's scientifically inaccurate.

". . . As a society we need to face the reality of it head-on . . . And despite its official protests to the contrary, the VA secretly agrees with me. Visit any VA hospital across the country and you'll see what I mean. What's the first thing you see when you walk in? A metal detector with an armed VA police officer standing nearby." (Morris & Plait, 2014)

I believe that David J. Morris makes a valid point. My understanding of 'Alternative Facts' is that they are lies! We face a massive problem that can no longer be swept under the carpet or falsely altered in the name of country and patriotism.

By facing it head on we can finally look into causation factors rather than chronically reacting to troublesome symptoms. Sweeping truths under the rug can no longer be tolerated. It's time for us to face the reality of PTS as a significant and enduring factor in the weakening of our military resilience and the undermining of family structure among those who serve or have served.

As described earlier, increasing numbers of our Veterans end up interfacing with the Criminal Justice System. Finally, an emerging awareness of their altered state and how it has manifested in antisocial behavior has led to the creation of the first Veteran's Court in 2008.

****

In 2007, Judge Robert Russell of Buffalo, New York, noticed that there were a lot of veterans showing up on his docket with addiction and mental health problems. He was having a hard time connecting with a particular Vietnam veteran.

The vet had his head down and was monotone in his answers. In a moment of exasperation, the judge said to a coordinator in the courtroom, who he knew had served in the military, "Can you take him out in the hall and talk to him, vet to vet?" Deutsch said.

After about 45 minutes, the two came back, and the judge called the case. The man was transformed.

He stood at parade rest with his head up and answered the judge with "Yes, sir" and "No, sir" and said he did want to be a part of the drug court program.

That's when the light bulb went off for Russell.

The judge worked with others in the court system and at the Veterans Administration to create a complementary program that would provide the usual elements of drug court plus military mentors to all veterans. Each vet would have a representative from the VA in court so they could get connected with services that would help. ("Drug-addicted veterans get 2nd shot at treatment court – CNN.com,")

****

We can only surmise what happened out there in the hallway of Judge Robert Russell's hallway. Perhaps the coordinator said something like: "Attention! Soldier, this is the best thing that's happened to you since you left the military. When you go back in that courtroom assume the proper respect to the judge. He's on your side. Dismissed!"

We can further imagine that through the fog and haze in this Veteran's mind, he recognized that he was again in a world that he was familiar with. Upon his return, the judge addressed him by his rank and name. And wow, the judge was standing there beside him, not up on his judicial bench.

At that point, he immediately recognized that he is speaking to someone from his own world. Perhaps security can come into his life again as it did while he was in service. He responds with, "Yes Sir!"

When he takes his seat, he notices that the Vet sitting beside him is called up for the presentation of a graduation coin. A Brigadier General who is visiting the court is asked by the judge to do the presentation.

Words are said that make this fellow stand proud. As he accepts his coin, a tear rolls down his eye. Our newcomer to the VTC is beginning to sense that this place is different. This place might be a better choice for him.

While it would seem logical for Veterans to choose a system that has an understanding of military culture, it also seems reasonable to check this question through a comprehensive inquiry. In other words, does the Veteran readily adapt to the military friendly atmosphere conveyed through the Veteran Court system?

Apparently, the answer is yes as discussed by the investigators in the following 2016 study. They explored this matter through interviews and focus group data noting that:

". . . it is imperative that the scientific community understand their operational procedures and assess whether they (VTC) are meeting a unique need beyond those addressed by other problem-solving courts.

"The results of this exploratory study suggest that a shared culture serves to motivate justice-involved veterans to seek out the veterans' treatment court over other treatment options and remain engaged in this problem-solving court, while inspiring a sense of obligation to do well in treatment for them and their fellow veterans.

"The shared experiences of military service and across-the-board support for fellow service members suggest that the veterans' treatment court creates a unique environment for pursuing treatment." (Ahlin & Douds, 2016)

Next, we must inquire as to whether the Veteran Treatment Court (VTC) does what it purports to do. One of the first attempts to formally study the issue of recidivism was done by comparing VTC participants with veteran non-participants.

A recidivism rate (repeated criminal offenses) of 66% was referenced for those judged through a traditional criminal court process. Taking this figure at face value, I take it to mean that only 34% of the Veterans who were judged in a traditional criminal court process were able to successfully avoid serving time in prison related to the charges they were facing. Additionally, these few avoided additional appearances within the context of the judicial system.

The authors of the following recent research study conclude that:

". . . The results of the current study reveal that VTC participants have lower recidivism rates and lower mean numbers of re-arrests than a similar group of veteran probationers, and these results are even more pronounced for VTC participants who graduated from the program." (Hartley & Baldwin, 2016). Because of the numerous findings within this study, I will paraphrase the important factors while crediting the authors.

The four groups in the study include the following: 1) VTC graduates; 2) VTC general treatment group; 3) terminated participants (dropped from VTC program due to non-compliance; 4) Control group (opted out of VTC program choosing traditional court proceedings).

Recidivism was defined as any new arrest subsequent to entering the VTC program for the treatment group and as any new arrest subsequent to the start date of their probation period for the control group. For ease of understanding, I will primarily be comparing the VTC graduate group versus the control group.

Regarding re-arrests, the VTC graduates had 18 as compared to 26 in the control group. Nearly half of the re-arrests for the VTC general treatment group came from terminated participants. Thus, only 9 of the graduated were re-arrested within the context of their program involvement.

The primary type of re-arrest found in all groups was Driving while intoxicated (DWI) suggesting that the issue of addiction is a primary factor in all groups. A finding of concern among the graduate group was an incidence of assault among 22% of the group.

From my perspective, the prevalence of incidents of this type reveal the ongoing nature of the underlying PTSD condition. This view was further supported by the finding at the 36-month point of 20% recidivism rates for VTC graduates.

While certainly this is a better figure than the 50% found in the control group, I believe that it can be lowered even more by addressing the causative factors that created the PTSD condition in the first place.

In summary, the recidivism rates for the comparison group are more than 1.5 times higher than the general treatment group and 2.5 times higher than the VTC graduates. (Hartley & Baldwin, 2016)

Comparing apples and apples, the study authors, through my understanding, mentioned a 66% recidivism rate for those adjudicated through a traditional criminal court process. The VTC 3-year graduates evidenced a recidivism rate of 20% for graduates, 31.7% for general treatment, and 50.0% for the control groups.

If I were that serviceman, I'd be weighing up to a possible 3-year tour in Judge Robert Russell's courtroom that seems to be a military friendly place with an 80% likelihood that I'd avoid re-arrest again and might have my record cleared for a new start in life.

I'd get to compare this with a 50% likelihood of being arrested again and having to serve jail time for each new charge if I choose a traditional court. My attorney thinks that I'll serve less time in the traditional court because he can plead my charges down. I think I'd sleep on it and hope that when I wake up, I'll make the right choice!

****

WARWICK, R.I. (AP) — William Delaney, a former Marine, had already served four years of probation for an alcohol-related offense in Florida and was back in court, this time in Rhode Island, for driving under the influence.

His newest brush with the law, combined with his alcoholism and depression, he feared, could close the door on the rest of his life.

That was almost two and a half years ago. Delaney now mentors other veterans in that same court, and he's working toward earning his master's degree in social work to continue helping veterans.

. . . Like Delaney, most of the 220 veterans who have completed the program haven't committed another offense. The rate of recidivism stands at about 6 percent, according to the court.

Today, there are more than 250 and hundreds more are planned, according to Justice For Vets, which advocates for the establishment of the courts and provides training for jurisdictions with new courts.

If they go to the veterans court, they have to follow whatever treatment the court prescribes to address substance abuse, behavioral or other issues and regularly check in with court staff, usually for 10 months to a year. At the end, often their case is dismissed entirely and expunged.

The court holds graduation ceremonies for veterans who complete treatment. . . The veterans were presented with a coin in the style of a military command coin, which is meant to show one's military affiliation and instill pride.

It bears the last six words of the Pledge of Allegiance: With liberty and justice for all. ("5 years later, Veterans Treatment Court is a success story,")

****

As noted in the Florida Courts webpage:

"Veterans courts are designed to assist justice-involved defendants with the complex treatment needs associated with substance abuse, mental health, and other issues unique to the traumatic experience of war. Some veterans returning home from war find it difficult to integrate back into the community.

"Veterans with untreated substance abuse or mental health illnesses, including those with post-traumatic stress disorder (PTSD) and traumatic brain injury (TBI), may find it even harder to return home, which can sometimes lead to criminal activity.

"Veterans courts involve cooperation and collaboration with traditional partners found in drug courts, such as the judge, state attorney, public defender, case manager, treatment provider, probation, and law enforcement.

"Added to this interdisciplinary team are representatives of the Veterans Health Administration (VHA) and the Veterans Benefit Administration- as well as State Departments of Veterans Affairs, Vet Centers, Veterans Service Organizations, Department of Labor, volunteer veteran mentors, and other veterans support groups.

"The most obvious distinction between a veterans court and other problem-solving courts is that it limits participation to current or former members of the military. Some of the other differences include the veterans court team encompassing at least one member who is familiar with veteran and military culture, terminology, benefits, and any other veteran or military issues that may arise.

"Veterans courts make use of the camaraderie that exists among all veterans. An essential part of veterans court is the addition of volunteer veteran mentors to assist their fellow veterans with a wide array of support. They are principal to the veterans court team and the participants.

"Their interaction with the participant, including a supportive relationship, maintained throughout the program, increases the likelihood that the participant will remain in treatment and improves the chances of success and sobriety.

"Veteran mentors volunteer their time and energy to assist their fellow veterans with peer support, housing, employment linkages, job training, education, transportation, disability compensation claims, discharge status and other linkages available at the local, state and federal level.

"Furthermore, the VHA plays a key role in veterans court as their services are provided to justice-involved veteran participants. Veterans treatment courts leverage resources available from the U.S. Department of Veterans Affairs to serve these offenders treatment needs." ("Veterans Courts," 2017)

****

As awareness about the toll of war on troops has grown and veterans of the recent wars in Iraq and Afghanistan have returned, the courts have gained in popularity. They rely on mentors, like Tim Wynn, who can easily relate to troubled military comrades.

Wynn, 35, who told his story in front of 1,000 people at the opening of the conference, said he was "deep into drugs and alcohol." He was arrested over and over, spent a total of a year in jail, lost his family and lost his mind.

"I was a maniac," he said.

Even after he got sober, he couldn't control a temper fueled by his experience in Iraq, etched in ink across his arms and invisibly in his brain, that would throw him into violent rages. But after a road rage incident where he attacked another driver and was charged with assault, he found himself in veterans court in Philadelphia. He finally got treatment for post-traumatic stress disorder, which had gone undiagnosed for more than a decade.

These days, Wynn occasionally finds himself in a crack house at 4 a.m. As a certified peer specialist, he's there to help a veteran whose predicament he knows well.

My clients are me two years ago" he said. ("Having veterans as mentors is key to treatment court success stories – Stripes,")

****

". . . Left untreated, mental health disorders common among veterans can directly lead to involvement in the criminal justice system. . . There is much documented evidence that a significant number of the Veterans who returned from the Vietnam conflict experienced rather severe problems adjusting to civilian life.

". . . An early sign that a Veteran may have unaddressed problems may be when they first break the law. The Veterans Court offers opportunity for the VA, local support organizations, and local communities to engage Veterans and offer treatment as an alternative to time in jail.

". . . The goal of Veterans Treatment Courts is to divert those with mental health issues and homelessness from the traditional justice system and to give them treatment and tools for rehabilitation and readjustment. . . Usually Veterans Courts hear cases involving misdemeanor charges . . . A Veteran's participation in treatment court is always voluntary.

". . . If the Veteran fails to meet the requirements of the program — for example, if he or she fails drug screenings or disobeys court orders — the Court will impose sanctions which may include community service, fines, jail time, or transfer out of Veterans Treatment back to a traditional criminal court.

". . . The Veterans Treatment Court model requires regular court appearances (a bi-weekly minimum in the early phases of the program), as well as mandatory attendance at treatment sessions and frequent and random testing for substance use (drug and/or alcohol)." (Absher,)

Based on Hartley and Baldwin's 2016 conclusions, above, it appears that the VTC treatment experiment is on the right track. What else comes out of their thorough analysis? Among the VTC participants, 18 re-arrests were recorded, 39% were charged with DWI's, public disorder charges were made in 28% of the participants and assault charges were made in 22%.

I can make a case can be made, based on these figures, that although the statistics are certainly an improvement as compared to the control group results, we can do better. There is a way to: 1) shorten the time involvement in the program; 2) diminish the number of those who drop out, 3) more rapidly reduce the number of re-arrests including some with serious charges.

I believe the way to do this is to turn off the **'kill switch'** in these returning warriors who have been unsuccessful in transitioning back to the civilian world. What seems to be a missing but crucial element in the VTC treatment regimen is the addressing of the **causative factors** that got the veteran into trouble in the first place.

My personal view is that: **although PTSD is triggered by trauma, it is really a disease of memory. The problem isn't the trauma; it's that the trauma can't be forgotten!** This new information is at the core of transformative opportunity for those who have suffered from the effects of PTS.

With break-through research now available, just the opposite of what the cynics and doomsayers are preaching can now be said with certainty. I dare to tell our veterans that hope is alive and that quite simply said: the 'fear switch' in your mind can be placed in the **off** position when it no longer needs to be turned **on**.

Although adjunct mental health services are available within the context of the Veterans Treatment Court, my perspective is that these adjunct services have generally proven themselves to be inadequate in fully remediating the effects that PTSD imposes upon the afflicted individual. This appears to be the weak link in the chain.

The continued need for elicit use of chemical agents has developed in the PTSD afflicted Veteran to vainly try to quiet the horrors that are trapped within him/her. Without going into too much detail, the following review of a number of qualified studies, referred to as a "meta-analysis', is considered to be a highly valid and classic assessment of the usefulness of 'gold standard' treatments. The authors report that:

"it is of particular concern that a recent review (meta-analysis) of randomized controlled trials conducted primarily among civilians reported that approximately two-thirds of patients who receive PET (Prolonged Exposure Therapy) or CPT (Cognitive Processing Therapy) retain their diagnosis post-treatment." (Steenkamp, Litz, Hoge, & Marmar, 2015)

The reasons that too many veterans self-medicate, act out in an anti-social manner, finds themselves at odds with the legal system, etc., is because their PTSD remains unresolved.

There is a known neurological pathway, definitively validated in an animal model, with emerging evidence for applicability to humans that provides us with a solid foundation to intervene in a remediation effort. Rather than using light, my treatment of choice is a sound-based, non-invasive procedure.

Finally, for humans, we have a non-invasive way to turn off the 'kill/fear/anger' switch. What might happen if this treatment intervention were added to the VTC program? I speculate that it would hasten the recovery process, diminish the dropout rate, and significantly reduce the re-arrest rate. Details of this treatment called RESET Therapy will be provided in the next chapter of this book.

Summary

I made the case that when Johnny comes home with PTSD, he is inclined to be hyper-aroused and overly sensitive to perceived intentions in others. With a disrupted sleep pattern accompanied by nightmares and flashbacks, he begins a downward slide by adding chemicals/liquids to the deadly mix. Unfortunately, for too many, this leads to isolation, homelessness, imprisonment, suicide and for some, homicide.

A history of the Veterans Treatment Court was provided with the elements that make it unique. Tentative and early research finding were provided supporting both the benefits and remaining mental health service deficits of the VTC system.

My primary objective in this chapter was to highlight the insidious nature of trauma as the primary causative element contributing to the Veteran's ongoing societal adjustment issues. Because of this factor, many require, either legally or illegally, the continued use of chemicals such as prescription cocktails that modify but do not eliminate troublesome symptoms.

I referred to current therapeutic interventions as failing in the total elimination of the full symptom features including sleep disturbance, nightmares and flash-backs. This deadly trio has proven to be resistant to all prior forms of therapeutic intervention. It took advances in neuroscience to finally understand the mechanisms involved that sustain these disturbing aspects of PTSD.

Finally, in the next chapter I will detail the nature of the 'healing sound' and how it alters the way that traumatic events are repeatedly restored in the brain. When this knowledge is provided with skill and expertise by a properly therapist, Johnny is finally freed from his 'protect and defend' status thereby permitting him to really and fully come home.

References

5, C. O., 2011, & Am, 3:08. (n.d.). Poll: 1 in 3 vets say Iraq, Afghan wars a waste. http://www .cbsnews.com/news/poll-1-in-3-vets-say-iraq-afghan-wars-a-waste/

5 years later, Veterans Treatment Court is a success story.http://bigstory.ap.org/article/f775b73

6315442ffaba933a72d84dcd3/5-years-later-
veterans-treatment-court-success-story

Absher, J. Veteran Treatment Courts http://www.
military.com/benefits/military-legal-matters
/veterans-treatment-courts.html

Ahlin, E. M., & Douds, A. S. (2016). Military
Socialization: A Motivating Factor for
Seeking Treatment in a Veterans' Treatment
Court. *American Journal of Criminal Justice*,
41(1), 83–96.

Booth-Kewley, S., Larson, G. E., Highfill-McRoy, R.
M., Garland, C. F., & Gaskin, T. A. (2010).
Factors associated with antisocial behavior in
combat veterans. *Aggressive Behavior*, *36*(5),
330–337. https://doi.org/10.1002/ab.20355

Drug-addicted veterans get 2nd shot at treatment
court-CNN.com.http://edition.cnn.com/2014
/08/26 /health/veterans-treatment-court/

From PTSD to Prison: Why Veterans Become
Criminals - The Daily Beast. http://www. the
dailybeast.com/articles/2013/07/28/from-ptsd-
to-prison-why-veterans-become-
criminals.html

Fulton, J. J., Calhoun, P. S., Wagner, H. R., Schry, A.
R., Hair, L. P., Feeling, N., … Beckham, J. C.
(2015). The prevalence of posttraumatic stress
disorder in Operation Enduring Freedom/
Operation Iraqi Freedom (OEF/OIF)
Veterans: a meta-analysis. *Journal of Anxiety*

Disorders, *31,* 98–107. https://doi.org
/10.1016 /j.janxdis .2015.02.003

Han, W., Tellez, L. A., Rangel, M. J., Motta, S. C.,
Zhang, X., Perez, I. O., ... Araujo, I. E. de.
(2017). Integrated Control of Predatory
Hunting by the Central Nucleus of the
Amygdala. *Cell,* *168*(1), 311–324.e18.
https://doi.org/10.1016/j.cell.2016.12.027

Hartley, R. D., & Baldwin, J. M. (2016). Waging
War on Recidivism Among Justice-Involved
Veterans: An Impact Evaluation of a Large
Urban Veterans Treatment Court. *Criminal
Justice Policy Review,* 0887403416650490.
https://doi.org/10.1177/0887403416650490

Having veterans as mentors is key to treatment court
success stories - Stripes. http://www.stripes.
com/having-veterans-as-mentors-is-key-to-
treatment-court-success-stories-1.360274

Lithwick, D., & Gilmore, D. (2016, January 5).
Prisons Have Become America's New
Asylums Slate http://www.slate.com/articles
/news_and_politics/jurisprudence/2016/01/pri
sons_have_become_warehouses_for_the_men
tally_ill.html

Morris, D. J., & Plait, P. (2014, April 17). War Is
Hell, and the Hell Rubs Off. *Slate.*
http://www.slate.com/articles/health_and_scie
nce/medical_examiner/2014/04/ptsd_and_viol
ence_by_veterans_increased_murder_rates_re
lated_to_war_experience.html

National Coalition for Homeless Veterans. http:/
/nchv.org/index.php/news/media/background
_and_statistics/

Profile of Veterans: 2009 - Post_911_ Veterans
_Profile_2014.pdf.https://www.va.gov/vet
data/docs/SpecialReports/Post_911_Veterans
_Profile_2014.pdf

Research on PTSD, Aggression, and Violence -
PTSD: National Center for PTSD. http://www
.ptsd.va.gov/professional/co-occurring
research_on_ptsd_and_violence.asp

Steenkamp, M. M., Litz, B. T., Hoge, C. W., &
Marmar, C. R. (2015). Psychotherapy for
Military-Related PTSD: A Review of
Randomized Clinical Trials. *JAMA*, *314*(5),
489–500.https://doi.org/10.1001/jama.2015.
8370

Street, 1615 L., NW, Washington, S. 800, &
Inquiries, D. 20036 202 419 4300 | M. 202
419 4349 | F. 202 419 4372 | M. (2011,
October 5). War and Sacrifice in the Post-
9/11Era.http: // www. pew social trends.org
/2011   /10/05/war-and-sacrifice-in-the-post-
911-era/

The new face of veteran homelessness, by Lily
Casura.https://www.tribtalk.org/2014/11/10/th
e-new-face-of-veteran-homelessness/

Veterans Courts. (2017, January 12). http://www.
flcourts.org/resources-and-services/court-im

provement/problem-solving-courts/ veterans-court.stml

Violence in Veterans, Fact or Fiction? http://www .pt sdupdate.com/violence-veterans-fact-fiction/

Wolfe, M. (2013, July 28). From PTSD to Prison: Why Veterans Become Criminals. http:// www. the daily beast. com/ articles /2013/07/28/ from-ptsd-to-prison- why-veterans- -criminals .html

Chapter Eight

A Special Sound That Heals

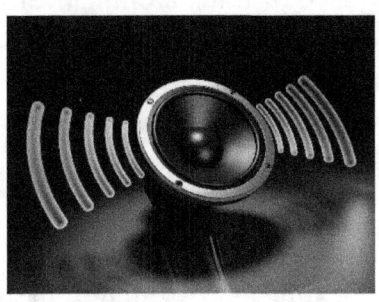

"Sound has a profound effect on the senses.
It can be both herd and felt.
It can even be seen with the mind's eye.
It can almost be tasted and smelled.
Sound can evoke responses of the five senses.
Sound can paint a picture, produce a mood,
trigger the senses
to remember another time and place.
From infancy we hear sound
with our entire bodies.
When I hear my own name,
I have as much a sense of it entering my body
through my back or my hand or my chest as
through my ears.
Sound speaks to the sensorium;
the entire system of nerves
that stimulates sensual responce."

Louis Colaianni,
The Joy of Phonetics and Accents

The plan for this chapter is to introduce you to a special and unique sound that is able to restore your loved one back to the person he was before the sudden experience of trauma dramatically altered his being. As part of this introduction, I will describe to you in non-technical terms how this amazing neuroscientific intervention works.

For some of you, this is not a surprise as sound has been used in various cultures for thousands of years as a tool for healing. For example, the drum is the oldest known instrument in the world, dating back to 4000 BC in Egypt. In my community, we have a weekly drum circle where people gather to share sound together.

By using rhythm and frequency as in our music, the human brain can down-shift our normal state of focus and concentration to that of a meditative state. This same concept is used in meditation by regulating the breathing frequency and depth of the breath.

Now I must confess my age of 77 because the newer forms of music that our youth prefer, such as hip-hop and hard rock, simply drives me crazy. Talk about the opposite effect of meditation! This form of music elevates my stress level, create imbalances in my nervous system, lowers my immunity and bothers my hearing. So, you can guess that I don't go to many hard rock concerts.

But you know what, my parents used to say the same thing when I first listened to Bill Haley and the Comets play "Rock Around the Clock" or Little Richard playing "Long Tall Sally." At any rate, when we are stressed, our entire relationship to sound changes. Everyday sounds distort or become magnified. Personally, when this goes on too long for me, I get migraine headaches.

A brief history lesson is in order here. In 1839 a Prussian physicist named Heinrich Wilhelm Dove, found that slightly different sound frequencies heard at the same time results in the brain producing a slightly different tone (frequency) that sounds like a beat.

Later, in 1973, Dr. Gerald Oster, a biophysicist presented a paper in Scientific American that documented how the brain is able to understand frequency signals and consequently produces a binaural beat effect. This happens when a tone is played in one ear and a slightly different tone is played in the other.

Keeping my non-technical promise in mind, a binaural beat is best understood literally as being able to hear two distinct sounds, one through each ear. This ability permits the individual to determine where the sound is coming from in three dimensions thereby permitting him to track moving sounds.

Finishing up my history lesson, a well-known Broadway musical composer (particularly to us older folk), George Gershwin wrote that, "Music sets up a certain vibration which unquestionably results in a physical reaction. Eventually the proper vibration for every person will be found and utilized" (Arem). Wouldn't Gershwin be pleasantly surprised to be aware that his predicted healing use of vibration is happening now?

What's important for you to know in this discussion is that the binaural beat comprises one essential corner of the change triangle that leads to the remediation of PTSD. As we proceed, I'll introduce the other elements. Also, at the end of this chapter I'll provide you with a transformative case example that puts it all together.

The next term I'd like to present to you is that of an 'emotional target'. This is an aspect of another corner in our treatment triangle that I'll fully describe as we proceed. At any rate, during the treatment, no talk takes place. All of the activity takes place within the imaginal ability of your Veteran.

Imagine that I'm asking your Veteran to select a trauma that maybe is at a 6 level on a 0 to 10-point scale. I explain that I would like it to be sensed as fully as possible in the body as well through smell, sound, visual recall, etc. I ask Johnny to avoid thinking about the target too much but that it's okay to do this to get the process started.

Now mind you, Johnny has been doing everything that's earthly possible to avoid what I'm asking him to do. I tell him that then when we do this correctly, he will only have to 'light-up' (activate) this target one more time.

Contrast this with a treatment they use at the VA called Prolonged Exposure Therapy (PET) where your Veteran talks about the worst trauma over and over again each and every visit with the counselor till he adjusts to it and he kinda becomes immune to it.

Or they might have Johnny do a thought based therapy called Cognitive Behavioral Therapy (CBT) where he's in a group with other vet's and they teach him how to think other thoughts about his PTSD to weaken its effects. It's kinda like learning how to talk yourself out of your nightmares and flashbacks.

The research on these two "Gold Standard" treatments suggests that perhaps one-third of the people who use it benefit from it. There is no research to suggest that the following PTSD symptoms are totally eliminated from these treatments: insomnia, nightmares, flashbacks.

They might also be considering providing Johnny with a 'medication cocktail' to try to control the symptoms because what he's already tried hasn't worked. However, his buddies that have tried it aren't like they used to be. Some of them call it the, "Zombie Effect."

The point being made here is that when Johnny learns from other Vets who were once skeptics and are now advocates, that this new type of treatment is not Bull S---, he's going to give it a thought. Maybe he's going to listen to a podcast of a Soldier that served 4 tours in Vietnam and has suffered from PTSD for 50+ years. This guy has become totally free of PTSD symptom after three treatments. Maybe he's going to think about this new treatment a little harder.

He might become concerned about his pension that he struggled so long and hard to get. He might remember the time when this condition wasn't even recognized. Wasn't there that film clip of General Patton slapping a Soldier who had 'shell shock.' Perhaps he's heard from so many that there is really no treatment to place this condition in complete and total remission. He's already heard others tell him that, "You just have to learn to live with it."

Well Johnny, this may have been true in the past because we didn't fully understand how trauma did this to you but now we understand. It gets intertwined into the memory system deep in your brain in a part that's right smack in the emotional center. Earlier we talked about how some music can really sooth you and other types can have exactly the opposite effect. In other words, music and emotion share many commonalities.

Back to the music. Music has wave lengths referred to as frequencies. When we tuned in the old-fashioned radios when I was a kid, the knob adjusted the frequencies to lock in the station. I bet not too many of you remember "The Shadow" or the kid's show, "Big John and Sparky."

Well, here's some good news for you. We can tune into the frequencies of trauma that are locked in our minds by attending to them rather than avoiding them. They too give off a frequency that is different from our other experiences. Almost like the screeching on the blackboard kinda sound. It gives you chills just thinking about it! This is the 'emotional target' I was talking about earlier.

As an extra freebie, other circuits besides the emotional one can also be tuned into. In my book, "PTSD Comorbid Conditions," I also list the following circuits: Addiction, Chronic Pain, Complex

PTSD, Dementia, Depression, Sleep Disorder, Survivor's Guilt and Traumatic Brain Injury. Six of the eight listed above can be utilized for treatment purposes through RESET Therapy. Dementia and Traumatic Brain Injury (TBI) are being looked at through other types of treatment.

Now if we had a way to adjust an external sound frequency to connect with (resonate) the emotional target, we've got two necessary components of our triangle of change in place. Tuning fork A and B illustrate the process. When you strike A, the vibration effects causes B to also vibrate. Notice that the term used is sympathetic vibration.

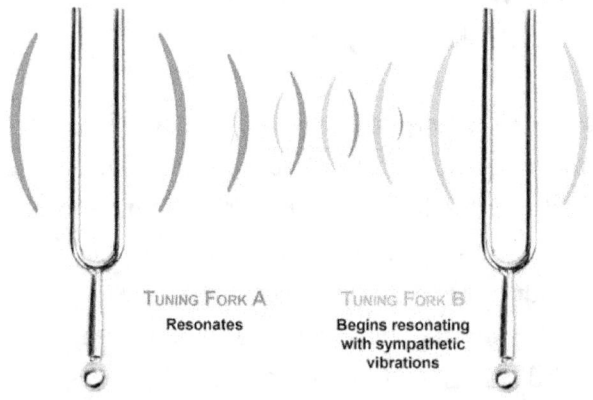

TUNING FORK A
Resonates

TUNING FORK B
Begins resonating with sympathetic vibrations

Treatment wise, I will set the binaural beat (two sounds heard as one in the brain) that resonates with an emotional target. This is the first step taken through which we can eliminate the emotional component of the PTSD condition. We now have the means to tune into the 'proper vibration' for each person and to use that frequency to resonate with selected targets.

As you know by now, binaural beats are created by sounds of slightly differing frequencies with each heard in one ear and the brain perceiving of them as one. This kind of neuromodulated sound has been proposed to induce relaxation, meditation, creativity and other desirable mental states.

At this point, let me introduce you to the Bio-Acoustical Utilization Device (BAUD) patented by Dr. Frank Lawlis and his son, T Frank Lawlis. Dr. Lawlis later developed numerous treatment protocols that remain in use today including the PTSD protocol being used in our current study. The Bio-Acoustical Utilization Device (BAUD) is a FDA class 2 accessory medical device designed to enhance brain plasticity in biofeedback programs. The term used for frequencies of sound beginning with one cycle per second is Hertz (Hz.). Thus, 60 Hz. equates to 60 cycles per second.

The BAUD creates sound waves from 39 to 362 Hz. that are heard separately in the left and right ears. The instrument consists of a handheld sound-emitting appliance that runs on batteries and is utilized by the patient in conjunction with a set of headphones. The

BAUD has independent volume controls for the left and right ears.

The device also has a tone (Frequency) Knob to adjust the sound frequency. It also has a "disrupter" adjustment which functions as follows: the tone generated in the left ear is presented to the right ear plus an offset based on the position of the Disrupter Knob. In other words, this final knob creates a different sound but the brain only hears it as one.

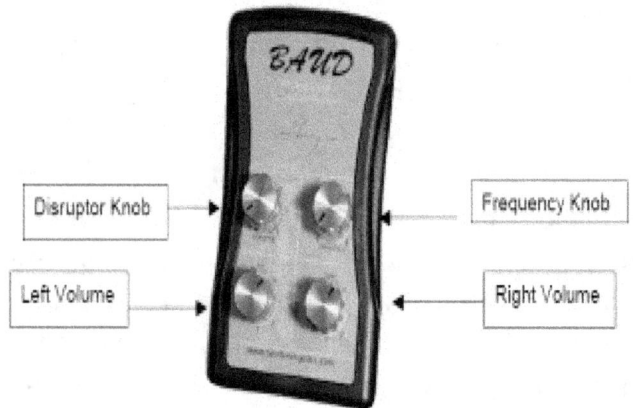

When the Disrupter Knob is set at the lowest level (0 Hz.), the frequencies heard in each ear will be exactly the same. At the other extreme, when the disrupter adjustment is at the highest level, (6) the tone heard in the left ear will be that of the right ear plus 20 Hz.

The BAUD and a good set of headphones are the tools utilized to make things happen. In some cases, hearing difficulties are present or the individual may be experiencing a ringing in the ears called Tinnitus. In such situations, I use a different headphone called a 'bone conducting' headphone that uses vibration to conduct rather than using sound. This works just as well and avoids making the ringing condition worse.

This is the point that I discuss the means through which the special sound (binaural) can remediate the PTSD symptoms. I've previously informed you that it is my belief that PTSD is a problem of the memory system.

Once it gets in this neuronal network where both memory and the emotions intertwine, it's hard to get it out. I've noted that talk alone won't do it and that repeating it over and over again messes too many people up.

I want you to understand the memory system a little better before I put the entire package together. With trauma, a package effect becomes stored in the emotional/memory circuits of the brain.

Some of it goes to the visual circuits, some to the muscles, others to the skin (kinesthetic) areas and so on. When something triggers this memory package such as a particular type of smell or sound, it may set the entire package off.

I'm often asked how this comes to be? If we look at evolution, survival of the species is a primary directive. I convey this by telling people that Mother Nature designed us to only smell the tiger's breath one time. In other words, if we survive that incident, Mother Nature wants to ensure that we don't go back for a second attempt.

Research into this area has produced repeatable results both in animal and human subjects. When this type of event occurs for the first time it is called **Consolidation**. After a period of time (some say up to a day or two) the trauma effect becomes locked into the system permanently. By the way, this process can also occur with positive memories as well. This is the way memory is placed in long-term storage.

An interesting aspect of this is that each time the trauma memory is triggered, it goes through another storage process called **Reconsolidation**. Now many researchers are involved in developing methods to intervene at this point that the restoration occur. Some inject medications, some use light, some are even trying it through the tongue. I use sound!

Why would so many educated folks spend so much of their time trying to alter this process? The answer is pretty straight forward. **If we can intervene at this crucial moment, the brain will restore the memory free of the emotional component.**

If you didn't get it the first time, let me say it again. The brain can change what it stores in the memory circuits if it's normal restoring process is interrupted. **Specifically, the emotional part of the memory can drop out!**

The following figure provides an overview of my perspective of the memory process. The first egg shaped illustration is labeled 'New Memory (active)' obtained through 'Learning' and Consolidated into the stored 'Inactive Memory' circuitry. When reactivated either intentfully or not, the memory becomes active again and subject to modification through varied forms of intervention including sound.

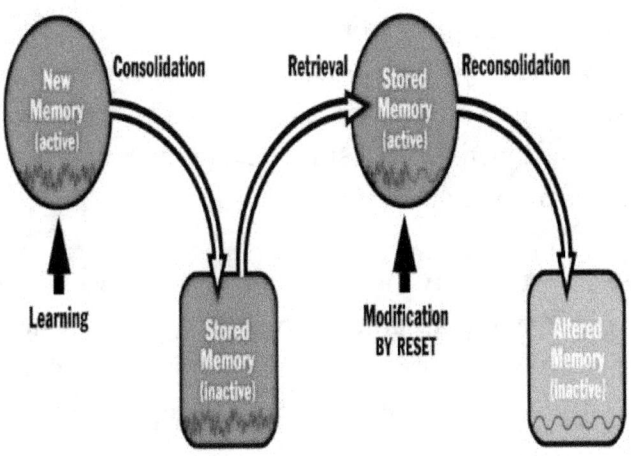

Learning generates a new short-term memory trace. The consolidation process moves it to long-term memory. Active or passive retrieval brings it back into short-term memory. This is the magic moment where change can occur before it is restored into long-term memory again (Reconsolidation). Note in the green box, the memory as illustrated in the wave form is now altered permanently.

In PTSD, the perceptual and emotional effects of this retrieval are highly disturbing. Reconsolidation of the memory occurs next. For a good or useful memory, this reinforcement or rehearsal can be beneficial. In PTSD, for the combat Veteran, First Responder and affected civilians, it is to be avoided at all costs.

To repeat, whenever a memory is retrieved, it can be modified through neuromodulation. The objective of RESET Therapy is to change the reconsolidation process. Clinical experience indicates that the process can be changed with positive results within 15 to 20 minutes of modulated sound (BAUD).

RESET Therapy is the treatment process that interferes with a targeted memory being restored repeatedly after it is selectively lit up in the emotional part of the brain through the patient's intentional focus. Wow, that's a mouthful.

The meaning of R-E-S-E-T follows: Reconsolidation Enhancement by Stimulation of Emotional Triggers.

This is what might occur in the treatment experience for Johnny. Perhaps he's already read something about what RESET Therapy is on my webpage: www.drlindenfeldresettherapy.com so he isn't coming in 'cold turkey.'

Johnny is asked to set the lower two Volume Knobs of the BAUD with his eyes closed. This is done to avoid his setting the dials by looking at the numbers rather than what is actually heard. I ask for a 'centering' of the sound in the mind. One could also call this a balancing of the sound between the left and right ear. The Volume Knobs can be adjusted one at a time or in unison.

At times, I will note a very high volume setting on one side as compared to the other. If this were the case with Johnny, I'd advise him to have his hearing checked. Occasionally, I'll come across an individual with hearing loss who will come in with hearing aids. I'll try the settings with the aids on and then off to get the best treatment option available for RESET Therapy.

Another option for those with extensive hearing difficulties is a bone conduction head set which operates through vibration rather than by sound. This supplement to the BAUD, assists patients with hearing problems, such as an individual who is deaf in one ear.

It would also be of use for those people who are sensitive to sound, such as those with sensory integration issues among autistic children or adults. Other clinic populations that would benefit from this tool will likely emerge as usage increases. Finally, I can imagine bone conduction headphones being used in RESET Therapy to further enhance the treatment effects by use of a different sensory channel that compliments and enhances the auditory channel.

Now we're ready to get serious by tuning in the binaural beat to properly resonate with the selected trauma/target. At this point I shift Johnny's attention to the upper dials of the BAUD. I will adjust the Frequency Knob (upper right) to a level where Johnny senses a connection (resonates) with the trauma. I have found in clinical practice that when the patient attempts to sustain focus on the trauma and simultaneously tune in the proper frequency, they will become distracted from their primary mission.

This aspect of the 'tuning in' process requires much expertise in order to get it right thus, this is not a do-it-yourself' type of project. If the frequencies are set improperly, failure is a certainty. My position on this matter is that our Veterans cannot be subjected to this therapy by improperly trained counselors who have not been Credentialed in RESET Therapy.

As the therapist adjusts the Frequency Knob, the patient is asked to 'light up the target' and to hand signal when maximum connectivity (resonance) occurs. The process involves adjusting the Frequency Knob slowly from 0 to 6 and then slowly backing it down to 0 to confirm the accuracy of the resonant setting.

When the patient's hand signal validates the frequency range, the setting is recorded for future use along with the volume levels. Now I must tell you that because some people have been exposed to horrendous trauma, their mind has disconnected the experience from their senses.

The psychiatric terms for this are disassociation, psychosomatic amnesia, etc. I refer to it as a disconnect. The memory is in the body but, the sensory experience is cutoff from the conscious mind. In other words, the individual is unable to sense when the sound frequency resonates with the trauma. This difficulty is addressed within my training program leading to certification for therapists.

The same sequence occurs with the Disruptor Knob with the patient hand signaling when the selected target begins to fade, become obscure, seem like an old picture, etc. What this means is that the proper settings have been found to change the restoration of the memory into its new form.

At this point, I initiate a five-minute trial asking Johnny to sustain focus on the selected target. After the trial, I ask what he experienced? I speak in terms of sensory awareness avoiding use of the words feel or think.

I have found that these words pull the patient away from the sensory aspect of the experience. Often the patient will come up with words describing what has just happened such as fading, diminishing, dwindling, disappearing, becoming foggy, or drifting away from the target.

I am inclined to stop the treatment at this point rather than proceeding immediately with a full 15- to 20-minute treatment session. I use the remaining time (if there is any) to have the patient check the target (the "switch" that triggers the symptoms) internally once again to re-evaluate the therapeutic intensity level.

I may later ask Johnny if his target changed or altered and if so, in what manner? I will suggest that he use a 0 to 10 rating scale with the 10 representing the highest intensity level possible. Thus, I would receive his subjective rating of the intensity of the target before and after the settings have been established.

Experientially, I've learned that my patients tend to fall into one of three groups. The first cluster experiences immediate relief ranging from partial to complete reduction of the targeted symptom. The second group notices a slight change initially that seems to build over the course of 24 hours. The third group, a minority, experiences no change at all.

I ask the patient to inform me of their response to the RESET Therapy the next day by phone, text or e-mail so that I can plan accordingly for our next scheduled session. With the first and second group, I proceed with full intervention when the next appointment occurs.

With the third group, I seek to clarify whether the target was fully lit up. Often, I find that the patient didn't understand what I mean by this due to a variety of factors. In extreme circumstances, as described earlier, I have found a dissociative disconnect that blocks the merging of material from the body and the mind. I've not run into a situation where it was not possible to find a creative way through the psychic wall, although I can imagine that this could occur.

When the full intervention session occurs, typically at the next scheduled appointment, Johnny will be asked to "run the script" internally for a full 15 to 20 minutes. More often than not, he will report that his inner mind took over from the script and ran its own agenda of nightmares, flashbacks, etc. When this occurs, I encourage this shift to the inner mind from the patient's conscious control efforts.

During the 'tuning in' trail and the full 15 to 20-minute treatment session, I remain busy. I'm carefully observing body signals, changes in breathing patterns and facial expressions while recording my observations within the context of the sessions.

One of my older patients came up with an awareness that her unconscious mind liked what was happening. She said: "Mikey likes it," referring to an old cereal ad that most of you young folk probably haven't heard of. However, I use this phrase to clarify the "letting-go" process, particularly for those who struggle to maintain whatever existing control they perceive they must still maintain.

Paradoxically, after 5 minutes or so, the annoying sound is reported by many to become increasingly comfortable. Some initially describe it as the sound of buzzing bees. We are universally and instinctively adverse to this type of sound. When asked later what had occurred, the patient typically notes a sort of dissolving or fading effect of the targeted material.

When asked after the treatment to discuss the target, the patient typically says something to the effect that he/she can recall with more clarity what happened at the time of the original incident but that the uncomfortable emotional component was gone. It is at this point that, usually, the patient's trauma can be conveyed verbally, fully and completely, rather than in the fragments that predominated before therapy.

This is the point where the angry cobra becomes defanged. If you've forgotten, one of my older Veterans told me that his PTSD was like having a p---ed off cobra with fangs ready to sink into anyone or anything that came close to it.

Following the full intervention session, I ask the patient to remain skeptical to the RESET experience and, as noted earlier, to call me 24 hours later to report any changes that may have occurred. Often, I receive positive feedback about a full night's sleep, none of the previous cold sweats at night, no anger outbursts at loved ones, no horrible flashbacks.

It still gets to me at an emotional level when I hear this. I feel as though I've facilitated someone's return from the brink. When you, as a family member, loved one, friend, etc., get to share this experience with your Veteran by sharing the changes in his demeanor, face, eyes and body, it's like your Johnny has finally come home.

You might begin to notice the 'old' Johnny being there again: his sense of humor; ability to understand things; comfort with people contact, etc. After the fear switch has been turned off, Johnny becomes the person he was meant to be before the trauma encounter. One fellow told me it was like his soul had returned to his body at the moment the demon left.

Finally, when this procedure is provided carefully by an adequately trained and certified therapist, Johnny's nightmares and flashbacks are finally, completely and permanently gone! You begin to sense the absence of the poison within him and begin to experience personally the elation and joy of participation in this process.

This becomes enhanced even further when the "thousand-yard stare" instantly disappears and is replaced by a look of wonderment and curiosity. This is the shift from 'protect and defend' to 'growth and exploration.' I assure you, this is a moment that you will never forget.

You have now been introduced to this incredibly effective treatment that can place PTSD into full and total remission. Others are trying to connect with specific areas of the brain such as the Limbic System by placing electrodes in the brain through invasive surgical procedures or ingesting Magic Mushrooms.

Contrast these approaches with their inherent risks with this non-invasive and safe form of intervention that is relatively free from side effects. By this I mean some minor buzzing in the ears may continue for a brief period of time after the treatment ends.

More often than not, when only one target is involved, it is necessary for the patient to go through this unique ordeal only one time in non-complex Post-Traumatic Stress Disorder. After experiencing rapid relief from this initial encounter, my patients tell me that they would have little hesitation to engage in the process again if a new target surfaces, and to do this as often as required to fully clear out any remaining remnants of trauma.

A case example will be helpful at this point to assist you to understand RESET Therapy from the perspective of a female Veteran who graduated from High School in 2002 and was inspired to serve in the military following 9/11/2001. She spent fourteen years in the Army beginning in 2002 including one tour in Afghanistan.

Her service took its toll on 31-year-old Military Police Officer. Sergeant First Class, Trudie Buchanan who noted that: "Being a victim of sexual assault in 2003 as well as being involved in an IED explosion on Christmas day 2005 caused emotional damage within me. I left the army last February, 2016 because the final straw for me was that I knew I was scaring my kids."

It was at this point that Trudie became aware that she had PTSD. While in service she noted that: "You don't really think about it because you don't have time. You have a mission. You have places to go and things to do. You're not encouraged to think about what you need because you're always focused on what others need."

While in service, this Veteran received the following decorations, medals, badges, citations and campaign ribbons: Afghanistan Campaign Medal with 2 Campaign Stars; Meritorious Service Medal; Army Commendation Medal (2nd Award); Army Achievement Medal (3rd Award); Army Good Conduct Medal (4th Award); National Defense Service Medal; Global War on Terrorism Service Medal.

Unfortunately, while in service, Trudie went through two failed marriages and was experiencing difficulty in her third. As typical for many females who serve, complaints of sexual abuse while in the military are either ignored or result in further disciplinary action taken against the individual who comes forth to complain. This was the case for Trudie who noted that: "After an investigation, my Company Commander and First Sergeant demoted me and took my money because I chose to report an assault."

Following the incident, Trudie began to self-medicate with alcohol leading to deterioration in her first marriage ultimately resulting in divorce in 2003. Her second relationship followed shortly after.

"We spent our first years of marriage apart. He was in Iraq in 2004 to 2005 and I deployed to Afghanistan from 2005 to 2006. During this period, I was still trying to process my sexual assault within the context of being deployed. Between us, over the course of six years, we had a lot of bad things going on. He finally left me and our divorce was final in 2009.

"I met my third husband in 2012. My alcohol use has subsided but I was still extremely stressed and anxious, easily angered with obsessive/compulsive tendencies. I felt the need to keep things in order because my life was so out of my control. It was very difficult for him to adjust himself to that. My interest in intimacy severely declined which further complicated my marital relationship. Clearly, I was on the road to another failed relationship however, children were involved this time.

"Early on, it was really easy to deal with my first child. She was just a baby and a pretty easy little kid. I went back to work after I had her but the stress continued at work. I became angry that I couldn't see her first steps and being around her during these first monumental points in her life.

"As she was growing up, I was becoming angrier and would take out the stress I was having on my husband. She would see us fighting when she was very little and it kinda continued on from there until I got pregnant with my son. Finally, we decided that I would leave the military because we were going to have two children and we didn't want to repeat the same process with my son."

Symptomatically, Trudie was experiencing difficulty with maintaining her emotional stability, manifesting irritability and explosiveness within her family and intimacy issues with her current husband due to her prior sexual assault.

She was experiencing nightmares one to two times per week and experienced flashbacks as well. She stated that: "It felt that I was yelling and no one was listening. I tried to avoid noises, crowed places and fireworks. I didn't watch military movies."

Trudie volunteered to participate in a study of 36-combat Veterans in the Sarasota, Florida region. She had become aware of this option through a picking up a brochure while visiting the MindSpa facility located in Sarasota, Florida.

She reported that: "With just one treatment, I was transformed into being the loving mom that my children needed. They're not feeling that same negative tension from me now so they're not reacting as negatively to my energy."

Buchanan said that RESET Therapy helped to reduce her everyday stress and totally eliminated her insomnia, flashbacks and nightmares. Within her first treatment experience, Trudie evidenced intense emotions stating that: "I felt like a ping-pong ball inside. Different triggers came up and I felt real heavy inside like my butt was made out of lead."

Prior to her second treatment experience, she reported that: "I just slept really well. I slept like a baby and I don't normally sleep that deeply or that well. On the night after the treatment, my sleep was amazing. My emotions were also subdued. I had a lot more patience with my kids but not with my husband yet. There is definitely a reduction of my depression and anxiety but I must confess that I have some reservations of what might yet come up with this treatment."

Because of her problematic history with males, Buchanan focused on male authority figures. She said: "The sound changed and then it smoothed out. My dad was there, angry and yelling. The sound then hop-scotched around with different pictures and images. It really felt good and the sound really changed."

In her third visit, she reported not experiencing any nightmares, flashbacks or insomnia over the past week. "Stress levels were much more even. Haven't had a screaming fit all week. I'm going to bed well even though the baby is teething. Still having intimacy issues with my husband due to my sexual assault and would like to change this problem."

Her RESET Therapy treatment focus on this difficulty. "It was more intense than the other stuff. I felt things – smelled things. I could smell the First Sergeant's office when I reported the rape."

Buchanan also was drawn by the 'healing sound' to focus on events that occurred while in Afghanistan. "I was doing a great deal of first aide intervention while there. It was like a tidal wave of emotion crashed over my head. In one situation, I couldn't get air support in quick enough to evacuate a wounded soldier.

"All of this altered with the sound. There were lots of things everywhere and I was seeing it, touching it. I almost lost a finger while I was there and it was hurting me. I remembered fighting with my ex-husband about it. He wanted me to wear my wedding ring and it hurt me to do so. While still listening to the sound, I sweated and had hot flashes – it was so physical. The sound wave would smooth out and then go to something else.

"Now, after only a few RESET Therapy sessions with Dr. Lindenfeld, it felt like the weight of the world was off my shoulders. It feels like I almost can't go back to where I was." Trudie has become an advocate for RESET Therapy participating in a TV segment on SNN News on February 23, 2017. You can view this brief portion of the show at: https://goo.gl/5OWu6B

EPILOGUE

A 2017 article in the European Journal of Psychotraumatology speaks to the societal components necessary for recovery from psychological distress after exposure to a traumatic event(s). The authors suggest that: "General social support, as well as support from a leader in one's working life, may facilitate enhancing social support from family and friends, as well as in work settings, may benefit those with psychological distress following a traumatic workplace event. (Birkeland, Nielsen, Hansen, Knardahl, & Heir, 2017)

Outside of the work environment, the phrase, 'It takes a village to raise a child' "may have its origins in the Bible, since it reflects a worldview regarding unity and self-sacrifice expressed in several passages of the Bible, such as Ecclesiastes 4:9,12 and Isaiah 49:15-16. This worldview is commonly seen in African cultures today.

"In many African communities, it is common for a child to be raised by its extended family, in many cases spending extended periods of time living with grandparents, aunts and uncles. Even the wider community sometimes gets involved, as children are seen as a blessing from God upon the entire community." ("What is the origin of the phrase "It takes a village to raise a child'?,")

Unfortunately, numerous factors have weakened the available support network including the deluge of pain medications that have flooded numerous communities across the nation. Within this context, "record numbers of Iraq and Afghanistan veterans have survived their war injuries and yet continue to experience pain and mental health problems, particularly posttraumatic stress disorder (PTSD).

"Little is known about the association of mental health disorders and prescription opioid use. Of 291,205 veterans who entered VA health care from 2005 through 2008, during 1 year of follow-up, 141,029 (48%) received at least 1 pain-related diagnosis. . . Of the 141,029 veterans with pain diagnoses, 15,676 (11.1%) received prescription opioids for 20 or more consecutive days; 77% of which were prescribed by VA primary care clinicians.

"This is the first national-level study to demonstrate that veterans of Iraq and Afghanistan with mental health diagnoses, particularly PTSD, are significantly more likely than veterans with no mental health diagnoses to receive prescription opioid medications for pain-related conditions. The association between PTSD and opioid prescription was robust because it was significant for all subgroups of veterans with PTSD.

". . . Veterans with mental health diagnoses prescribed opioids, especially those with PTSD, were more likely to have comorbid drug and alcohol use disorders; receive higher-dose opioid regimens; continue taking opioids longer; receive concurrent prescriptions for opioids, sedative hypnotics, or both; and obtain early opioid refills.

"Finally, receiving prescription opioids was associated with increased risk of adverse clinical outcomes for all veterans returning from Iraq and Afghanistan, especially for veterans with PTSD, who were at highest risk of alcohol-, drug-, and opioid-related accidents and overdose, as well as self-inflicted injuries." (Seal et al., 2012)

Doctors in the United States began prescribing opioids — powerful narcotics that include pill-form painkillers such as methadone, oxycodone and hydrocodone — to treat pain at unprecedented rates in the 1990s. The medical community adopted the practice more commonly despite long-standing fears that the drugs would lead to addiction, mostly as a result of promises from pharmaceutical companies that their products were safe treatments for pain. . . by 2015, deaths due to opioid overdoses surged to about 62 a day, according to the Centers for Disease Control and Prevention. ("The opioid epidemic could turn into a pandemic if we're not careful - The Washington Post,")

Unfortunately, with increasing levels of stress in our society, the impact on the primary socialization entity, the family, has become profound. This is further magnified among those who serve to protect us, whether abroad or at home.

Over the course of writing a number of books, my perspective of PTSD has altered. I have come to view this condition as being equivalent to a computer virus that enters the family network through a primary carrier. Once in the system, progressively and insidiously, growth processes ebb while the virus infiltrates and distorts the potential of all of those involved.

At the core of my perspective about PTS is the belief that we can reset the neuronal network that produces the symptom picture that Johnny brings home with him. Within this context, there is no need to call his condition a 'mental illness.' Rather, I fully believe that we can directly intervene and alter the causative agent that resides in the memory system in the brain called the amygdala.

To document this phenomenon, my colleagues and I are embarked on a major study of 36-combat Veterans in the Sarasota, Florida area. We plan to submit the results to a peer reviewed journal as our next step towards broader acceptance of this treatment which I refer to as RESET Therapy.

I end this discourse by assuring those families struggling with a loved one who has PTS that lasting relief is possible. I've provided you with a journey that took you through varied aspects of the PTS condition sharing stories of both failure and success.

A number of my own patient's case studies were included in order to diminish the mystery surrounding the use of binaural sound. Please let others know about what you have learned so that may also come to have hope once again.

In closing, I'd like to once again invite you to visit my webpage for further detailed and comprehensive information at: www.drlindenfeldresettherapy.com. At this site you will find blogs, published articles, additional books, media examples, treatment options and much more. Finally, please consider adding a review of what you think about this book when you complete it.

George Lindenfeld, Ph.D.
Diplomate in Clinical Psychology

References

Seal, K. H., Shi, Y., Cohen, G., Cohen, B. E., Maguen, S., Krebs, E. E., & Neylan, T. C. (2012). Association of Mental Health Disorders With Prescription Opioids and

High-Risk Opioid Use in US Veterans of Iraq and Afghanistan. *JAMA*, *307*(9), 940–947. https://doi.org /10.1001/jama.2012.234

The opioid epidemic could turn into a pandemic if we're not careful - The Washington Post. https://www. washingtonpost.com/news/in-theory/wp/2017/02/09/ the-opioid-epidemic-could-turn-into-a-pandemic-if-were-not-careful/?utm_term=.5f05f9609a2e

What is the origin of the phrase "It takes a village to raise a child'? https://www.reference .com/ education /origin-phrase-takes-village-raise-child-3e375ce098 113bb4